The Nightingale Gene

# The Nightingale Gene

Jayne Van Brunt

NEW YORK

LONDON • NASHVILLE • MELBOURNE • VANCOUVER

# The Nightingale Gene

## Lessons to Living a Balanced Life and Having the Nursing Career of Your Dreams!

Published in New York, New York, by Morgan James Publishing in partnership with Difference Press. Morgan James is a trademark of Morgan James, LLC. www.MorganJamesPublishing.com

The Morgan James Speakers Group can bring authors to your live event. For more information or to book an event visit The Morgan James Speakers Group at www.TheMorganJamesSpeakersGroup.com.

ISBN 9781642790269 paperback
ISBN 9781642790276 eBook
Library of Congress Control Number: 2018937270

**Cover Design by:**
Christopher Kirk
www.GFSstudio.com

**Interior Design by:**
Chris Treccani
www.3dogcreative.net

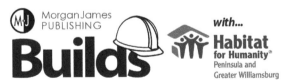

In an effort to support local communities, raise awareness and funds, Morgan James Publishing donates a percentage of all book sales for the life of each book to Habitat for Humanity Peninsula and Greater Williamsburg.

Get involved today! Visit
www.MorganJamesBuilds.com

# Table of Contents

# Introduction

M arie stepped off the plane in a fog following her virgin eighteen-hour flight to Italy. She stayed awake the entire time, watching movie after movie, while the plane took her further from her chaotic life. She was all set to keep up with work during the three-week trip, had programmed her phone so that she could get voicemail every day, and would check email on her work computer every night. Why did she agree to take work with her, seriously? *Because I never say no to him, that's why*, she thought. The movies were a mild distraction to the work she had left behind. She hoped a break from the hospital would make her relax but she doubted anything would.

It wasn't the best time to take off and her manager was not happy she would be gone for that long. She was feeling guilty about it too, but this was the first time she had ever been gone for more than a week and she was ready for a break. The job had become more stressful with the merger. She was finding it harder to take a deep breath, and tried more often to relax with a glass of wine or two right after work. Right after work was sometimes early afternoon and it worried her that lunchtime didn't seem that unreasonable some days either.

It was September 2006 when she set foot in Florence. She would turn 45 a month later. The tour van picked her up along with the large box that held her shiny new custom-made bike and two canvas bags full of multiple changes of clothes, three cycling jerseys and shorts, make-up, hairspray, curling iron, and the other necessities she required to live each day. The bags were much heavier than she remembered, and she struggled to get everything to the curb for the pick-up. She was embarrassed when she noticed how much more stuff she had than the other passengers and would continue to feel that way every time her baggage was carried up flights of stairs by the tour guides in the many hotels they would stay over the course of fifteen days.

Everything around her was strange as the van departed the Aeroporto di Firenze and headed the 8 km into the city. The cars, buses, and taxis were miniature versions of similar models she was used to seeing at home, but there were more scooters and bikes on the main roads. All of them mingled so closely together on the narrow cobble stone streets, managing to go much faster than seemed safe. It made her anxious watching them, imagining the impending crash she was sure would happen any second.

She was so tired, a different kind than she had ever known. She would later describe to friends back in Seattle that the *jet lag* made her more exhausted than she remembered being after both kids were born, even worse than doing night shifts at the hospital during her first job as a nurse. She was all turned around and wanted to sleep the days away in the dark hotel room, and would have if her husband hadn't forced her out of bed.

The bike tour would start in two days, so her only chance to see Florence was now, he had begged. Little did she know he had planned the whole trip, complete with tours of the Galleria dell' Accademia where Michelangelo's David stood, the Cathedral, the Museo Galileo and the Uffizi Gallery.

The first afternoon after being pulled from a deep sleep, she pouted as they left the hotel to take a walk. He steered her around a corner and into the Piazza Della Signoria and stopped abruptly. The shock of what lay before her jolted her awake. She had never imagined the ancient beauty of such a place and as she began to take in the larger-than-life statues, the alabaster columns, and the twenty-foot bronze doors filled with intricate engravings at the entrance of the cathedral, tears flowed down her cheeks. This was nothing like the Bellagio in Las Vegas, nothing like the many places she had travelled in her mind while reading books and watching movies.

They walked hours each day, crossing the Ponte Vecchio, opening heavy old doors that led to limestone floors and centuries-old church pews, where they would sit in the quiet and stare at the stained-glass windows and fresco paintings. She would never forget holding hands as they sat at the back during the evening concert in the quaint Santo Spirito church which happened by accident after walking in that day and being invited to return.

There were other delicious memories that she would return to as the years passed. The food and wine somehow tasted so much better than at home, giving her ideas about the new meals she would create for friends, knowing the perfect food would somehow make every night more enjoyable. She wondered if she could even find boar or goat for a ragu and how did they make the sauce so rich?

Florence would come back to her often the first few years, like an old friend. Certain moments would take her back in a flash, like watching her husband's hands as he tossed the homemade pasta in the flour to keep it from sticking while making dinner for friends. She would tell him how much the veins in his hands, the muscles in his arms, the way his fingers curled slightly reminded her of David. She would love him more for the precious memory.

They left Florence to begin the first of many bike trips in Italy and France they would take over the next several years, but the tour of Tuscany would remain in the deepest part of her heart where gratitude resides. She would often give thanks to her husband for taking her on that very first trip and for planning the many trips that followed. She would admit that if it hadn't been for him, she would not have had the courage to travel overseas. He would disagree and tell her nothing was braver than leaving a small town to go to college far from her family, and that she must have always had the desire and strength to get away. She feared he didn't really know her after all.

She would dream of that first trip and the promises she had made to herself to be different once she was back home. She would pay more attention to those she loved and she would slow down. She would use the beads she bought in Florence to design something special to wear to remind her of the small shop she found that sold iridescent glass beads. She would live more balanced like the Italians do, taking their late afternoon family time while the shops are closed. Even tourists there were expected to relax for a few hours and so they did, the quiet lulling them into an afternoon nap or a much anticipated read.

But there was a voice she rarely allowed herself to entertain, speaking a truth that she wasn't ready to accept. She wanted to live differently – her heart was pulling her back to the quiet in

Italy – but she didn't know how. Her life was like a train out of control and she had no idea where the brakes were. She often felt anxious, her heart racing as if she was the train heading over a cliff.

Despite her best intentions, work outpaced any efforts she made to get control of her life. Deep down she knew, if she was to live this balanced life, to be this creative woman she desired, her job had to change. The job that allowed her trips to Europe, more independence than she had ever thought possible, and enough challenge to keep her engaged was perfect. So why did this nagging voice continue to force her attention?

She knew the job was stressful but what nurse didn't experience stress? She often worked twelve-hour days but she was managing everything just fine. She could make this work if she tried a little harder to keep everything organized. She would spend more time cooking and doing jewelry. She would take better care of the house, enjoy the kids, and love her husband more often.

And she did for a while. Every trip away from her normal routine felt like an injection of inspiration that transformed her for a few weeks. But then, just like a drug, the feelings wore off and she was back to her old self, caught up in the firestorm that was her life.

I met Marie at a nursing conference the summer of 2016. She described in vivid detail the many trips she had taken with a smile on her face, but her eyes spoke regret. She was tired from the long hours she was putting in at work and the stress showed. Her face relaxed a bit as she talked about the cooking classes she had taken in Lucca, the beautiful kitchens they had used in the VRBO houses they rented in Provence, and the jewelry she used to make, but there was something in the way she talked about her many adventures as if they were part of her distant past. They were memories she could easily recount, but the pain was obvious in her voice, the tears now brimming over despite her best efforts to stop them.

She had recently made a lot of changes that she hoped would give her more time to do the things she had always said she would do. The new position was supposed to relieve some of the pressure, but instead the stress was even more evident. She described the imbalance in her life by talking about her chaotic thoughts: *It's as if there are competing voices in my head, fighting for my attention and I just want them to stop. I don't sleep well, and I cry easily over the slightest comment anyone makes that reminds me of everything I haven't accomplished, the promises I broke to myself.*

She found less joy in biking, wasn't inspired to cook anymore, and spent more time at work than ever before. When she was home, it felt like a stranger's, like she was imposing on someone else's life. She doubted herself more and wasn't even sure she wanted to leave her job. If not this job that she had known for over two decades, then what? What could she do to fill her days, to make a living? It would be irresponsible for her to make a big change that would impact them financially. She refused to listen to her husband telling her they would be fine. It angered her to even talk about the option, so remote was the possibility that it sounded crazy.

I recognized the struggle Marie was having. *No* was not a word in her vocabulary. She was more than competent in her job and, because of that, was often given extra work to do. There was a time when that would have given her great satisfaction, but she couldn't remember the last time she felt fulfilled. She was trying to be someone that everyone expected her to be, the person she had led everyone to believe she was. The constant battle with herself was taking a toll.

The nurse in me wanted to prescribe something in the form of immediate transformation, but I knew – much like her injections of inspiration from the trips she had lived – there was no quick fix. I turned to Marie, so our eyes connected, and told her a story about a woman who reminded me so much of her. A woman who struggled for years to find balance. I showed Marie a new perspective and a way to sort the many voices that caused chaos in her life, so she could make a clear and confident decision about the next steps with her career. She would decide if she should stay or go, but she would no longer run away from the decision as she had done for years.

# Chapter 1

# Tipping The Scales

*"You can't start with imbalance and end with peace,
be that in your own body, in an ecosystem or between a
government and its people. What we need to strive for is
not perfection, but balance."*
**–Ani DiFranco**

Nurses are caregivers by definition, destined to a life of serving others without question, nor desiring to do anything else. Nurses are not the only ones, as more demand is being placed on family members, especially women – daughters, sisters, wives, mothers – to provide care in the home to a very sick and taxing population. There are many women I work with who say that while they don't have a degree in nursing, they often play the role. It takes a special person – nurse, designated nurse, or caregiver – to balance this calling while remaining intact, their own needs barely discernable from the most obvious in front of them. You are the Nightingales, one and all, part of a distinct breed that must learn to find balance to survive. But how does one remember to give care first to themselves when there is so much to do for others?

I began writing this book over a year ago following a women's leadership retreat in Hawaii. This was the first time I could remember spending time focused only on what I imagined doing next in my life, removed from the daily stresses, free from the multitude of decisions that had to be made. The journal entries I made, while attempting to answer the questions asked at the retreat, morphed into the beginnings of a book about my life as a nurse, past, present, and future.

"Who is this woman who has achieved so much?" was a question that I struggled to answer. "Who am I now, and is this it? Isn't there more I have to offer in this fall season of my career and life?" I was grateful for the nursing degree that allowed me so much flexibility in my career, but I was worried too. I had been out of nursing school for more than thirty years, and realized the issues that sent me away from bedside nursing still existed today, but in a far more dramatic a fashion.

Nurses were leaving their jobs, and often the profession altogether, citing forced and unplanned overtime, poor management, and unsafe working conditions due to a high patient to nurse ratio. We had done little to move the profession beyond an hourly blue collar job, and women (being the majority), were choosing higher pay and more flexible schedules that supported better work-life balance for their families.

Every day, I interacted with nurses that were voicing their concerns about the profession they loved, including their fears that before long, the short staffing issues would become paramount, continuing the vicious cycle that forced nurses away in the first place.

"Who is this woman…?" "A nurse," was always the first thing I said. First and foremost, born, bred, and proud, I am part of the tribe of the Nightingales, the nurses who focus on the care of individuals at their most vulnerable. The profession that takes an oath to protect, advocate, and promote healing to those in need; to support their families and communities with the utmost respect and deference to their beliefs should their loved one die while in our care. Charles Dickens said a nurse must: *Have a heart that never hardens, a temper that never tires, and a touch that never hurts.*

Nightingales carry a rare gene, the insatiable desire to care for others while ignoring their own needs. It is both a superpower and a poison, the unlimited amount of empathy pointing outward, in one direction, with no ability to ask for or seek anything in recompense. In their true desire to serve each patient, nurses give a piece of themselves without question, experiencing the gift of another life, exposed and fearful, seeking comfort and guidance. Barely noticed, the small chinks in the armor of the Nightingales begin to weaken them to the pain and suffering of others in a way that is not easily diminished by the sweetest of life's distractions. To have a heart that never hardens is to have a heart that is constantly exposed and easily bruised.

The dilemma nurses face is not easily resolved. The work is hard physically and mentally, taking a toll on even the strongest. It is time to accept care, Nightingales, from anyone or anywhere you can. We have spent a lifetime giving everything to others and that is as rewarding a calling as anyone can find. But without taking care of ourselves, there is the real possibility of extinction.

This is a profession for the brave and strong, but also for the smart. Healthcare offers so many options for ambitious nurses and, in some cases, these choices lead them away from the hospital setting, or out of the profession. Hospital bedside nursing may be the most rigorous, but the high level of stress can be found in all positions, inpatient or out.

I wasn't close to entertaining the idea of retirement, but the thought of continuing to do the same thing for another twenty years made my head spin. I was exhausted by the work, yet continued to take every opportunity to be with the team, meeting patients, helping. I knew my health wasn't great, but I was too busy to make exercise and eating right a habit that stuck for more than a few days at a time. I began to have doubts about my ability to physically and mentally continue what I was doing. Some days I felt the panic swell up in me to the point that I struggled to catch my breath. I was back and forth like a ping-pong ball: Today I hate my job, yesterday I loved everything about it.

I did a lot of things to ignore my deepest fears – the ones that would surface in the middle of the night. *I won't survive if I stay, I will be lost if I go. What am I going to do if not this?* The retreat set this book in motion, but the answers to the questions had been years in the making. A life transition was afoot, creeping up on me slowly, like the faucet drip you barely notice until the stillness in the house amplifies the sound to an annoying splash, one you can no longer ignore, and one that will not be silenced without physical effort.

Lifetime Nightingales, you've known a career that has been spiritually rewarding, mentally taxing, and physically exhausting. How can you find the energy required to support new nurses? If you're not up for the job, who will be, and what will happen? The dilemma is hard to reconcile. Young ones today, who believed nursing was a perfect profession and graduated with joy in their hearts only to find weary and burned out nurses, please find the courage to hang in there, to seek compassion in your managers and mentors, to demand an environment that is healthy for you and the patients.

There is hope that we *lifers* will return to show you the way. We know what you need to grow and to thrive as happy nurses who nurture happy patients. We know that without a strong mentoring program and a supportive network, you will flounder, bounce around between units, take a different job in another setting, or leave the profession altogether. A study in 2014 stated that new nurses remain in their jobs less than two years and cite two primary reasons for leaving: poor management and burnout. We know change is inevitable if you are to survive, and we need you.

Take care, Nightingales. This profession is not for the faint of heart. We are hard wired to care for others while putting our own needs on the back burner. We learn to suck it up, hold back the tears, and teach our new grads to be tough, or find something easier to do. Thirty-two years after graduating from nursing school, I still hear the phrase *nurses eat their young* and found several books on the topic. I might have had the same frightening, bully experiences at the age of twenty-two, somehow being devoured once I started working in a hospital, but looking back now, that was far from the truth.

I experienced only kind, solicitous oversight from mentors who taught me to observe everything, miss nothing, and always show compassion even in the hardest of times. These women cared for me, sheltered me from the rages of doctors, and made sure I didn't harm a patient, ever. Do nurses eat their young, or do they protect them and their patients with wary supervision? We might have been too old to walk onto a busy street only to be killed by a car, but we could have done serious damage to a patient if not for the nurses keeping constant vigilance.

The fact that this is more than tribal knowledge today astounds me. In one blog post I read recently, the young graduate was already preparing for a fight during orientation on his new unit. Have we not accomplished anything in the decades this profession has existed? It is possible we've gone backward. Is it true that we don't give our young a fighting chance? It is possible the nurses remaining to help are too burned out to care. Is there no fun to be had in this profession, still as serious as Florence in the trenches? Yes, it is quite possible we still have problems, Nightingales, if what I've read is true. But there is hope in a better future, if we all work together.

Three years ago, there were an estimated 3.7 million nurses in the U.S. Ninety percent were women, more than fifty percent were over the age of forty, and 165,000 were new grads. By the year 2020, the U.S. estimates a workforce shortage of 1.5 million nurses, half from baby-boomer nurses retiring and half from the twenty percent increase in demand expected from the aging population. In a study from 2014, sixty-six percent of the nurses age fifty-five and older stated the quality of care had declined and many were looking to find other career opportunities to allow them to retire early; the rest would remain where they were until retirement.

More than 500,000 wise and tenured nurses are either sticking it out in their current jobs, burned out and waiting for retirement, or they've found alternate careers that fit for them but have little impact in mentoring younger nurses in desperate need of experience. There are not enough nurses to replace those who will retire, yet new grads are finding it difficult to get experience. In a study from 2012, more than one third of the new grads entering the work force from four year degree programs were unemployed four months or longer after graduating because most hospitals require a minimum of two years' experience. In California, 60 percent of the new grads are unemployed.

We have the supply – there is demand – now the call to action. Nurses everywhere, you have so many choices to find a job that fulfills, to demand a perfect fit for you. In a review of more than fifty hospitals, I found positive stories of the impact nurses are making on organizational change. Hospitals are listening to the demands nurses are voicing, and managers are reacting to the serious retention issues and putting into place better working conditions, less overtime, flexible schedules, and perks that extend beyond salary.

Over eighty percent of the nursing positions in healthcare and almost one hundred percent of household healthcare decisions are managed by women, yet we continue to hold less than ten percent of the executive level positions and get paid less than men in the same positions. We have a history of lacking empowerment, of deferring to doctors, of standing up for patients but not ourselves.

Soledad O'Brien put it this way: "The journey is valuable, but believing in your talents, your abilities, and your self-worth can empower you to walk down an even brighter path. Transforming fear into freedom – how great is that?" There are so many opportunities for women with nursing degrees to make a difference and it takes finding a fit that allows balance in your life, trust in yourself, and the ability to push past fear.

I am old enough to understand that a healthcare crisis exists today and – despite intelligent and powerful people taking a stab at it – we continue to struggle. We face serious and complex issues that are not easily resolved. But change is possible and will happen by taking baby steps forward. I wrote this book as a tribute to caregiving and nursing – a profession comprised of mostly women – and it will be those women, young and old, who will drive the efforts in healthcare. But only if burnout is kept in check.

Sometimes a change in thinking is all we need to breathe life into our careers. Sometimes, the comparison of what you love about your job and what's available to you offers the ability to consider clearly your choices. If you are deciding to stay in your current position or to go; if work-life balance has been a struggle and you're wondering if you can keep managing your schedule without crashing; if you're considering a change of any kind, this book will give you food for thought and some tools to make your decision with confidence.

The lessons in the book are about finding balance in a profession that demands so much of the very kind of people that desire only to care for others. It is possible to get lost in the process of caregiving, but also possible to find balance again. I will teach you ways to spin the thoughts that hold you back in order that you can move forward, to take time to simmer and to journal your best experiences, and finally, to devise a year-long plan that allows you to soar in the career that fits you perfectly. Let's get started!

# Chapter 2

# The Work-Life Dilemma

*"There is no such thing as work-life balance. Everything worth fighting for unbalances your life."*
**—Alain de Botton**

One only needs to do a search for the words stress, work, life, and balance to find all kinds of warnings about what happens when there is an unequal load. Nurses are taught about the effects of chronic stress on the body. They know that it's critical to pay attention to the symptoms of stress and to protect themselves from the imbalance that can occur when putting others first. Instructors warn caregivers to be careful, because without boundaries, their need to keep a constant vigil can lead to uncontrolled stress and illness. Nurses may know better than family members that stress can be disastrous, but rarely consider the effects it might have on their own bodies.

In an article by Cynthia Orange, she mentions, "The paradox of choosing to practice empathetic compassion is that such an act has the potential to fill you up both emotionally and physically or suck you dry." It's important to learn to be your best caregiver self, respecting your own and others' boundaries, while maintaining intention and self-awareness. Imbalance occurs when you over-commit, without thinking it through, saying yes even though you already have too much on your plate, then later regretting you did not make better choices for yourself. I learned the hard way what happens when you ignore the signs.

We had a New Year's Eve party leading into 2011 and I had a high fever. My son and husband had already had the same symptoms and I pushed away their claims of how bad it was, secretly thinking all men are babies. I could handle the cooking, cleaning, and entertaining even if I was so sick my head was spinning every time I moved too quickly. Retiring to bed was not an option even though it was offered by everyone. There was no way I was going to miss the party I planned and looked forward to all week.

Two days later, I was in the clinic because my legs were tingling, and I couldn't ignore the siren in my head that something was wrong. The clinic confirmed I had a bad cold, pneumonia, and sinusitis but before I left I asked again about the legs. That can happen with an overwhelming infection, the nurse claimed. Despite my knowing better, I was relieved that I could go home and rest up with my drugs and Nasi-pot and I'd be better in a couple of days. Whew, crisis averted, I thought.

I sent my husband on a ski trip with friends that would take him four hours away. I would join them in a couple of days once the drugs kicked in. Two days later, I was sicker than ever, so weak I didn't think I could get out of bed, but so thirsty and struggling to breathe that I wanted to get to the first floor for tea and a shower. I made it down the flight of stairs but changed my mind at the bottom. The first couple of steps back up the stairs were hard, but I convinced myself it was because I was so weak. The next step didn't happen. I couldn't force my leg to lift off the step.

I grabbed my car keys and drove to the ER. Within two hours, I was throwing up and in so much pain I couldn't stay still despite the narcotics they'd already given me. "We think you have multiple sclerosis but need to do a spinal tap to be sure," said the ER doctor. The rest is a blur, husband and friends showing up in the ER, drug haze, so much pain, then sleep, then back awake with pain. I was admitted to the cardiac unit because my blood pressure and heart rate were crazy high and because there was no diagnosis yet.

A week went by remembered only in flashes: My husband sleeping in a cot, demanding more pain medication, asking the nurses to please be quiet so I could sleep, more pain than I had ever experienced, my spine and legs feeling like a rotten tooth or earache at their worst. Other events I forgot completely, like friends coming to give me a pedicure, one eye covered with a patch, the other frozen open.

I was moved to rehab after the first week. I couldn't talk, walk, or swallow yet, but was more aware of what was going on because an angel in the form of a neurologist recommended a drug commonly used to treat seizures, for the nerve pain. With Guillain-Barre Syndrome (GBS), the autoimmune disease I had, the body doesn't recognize good cells from a virus, and begins eating away at the muscle sheath wrapped around the nerves that make up our peripheral nervous system. It is the number one cause of acute paralysis in America.

GBS usually starts from the ground up, with the first symptoms being tingling in the feet and legs. The progression from tingling to paralysis can happen in a matter of two days to a week. In emergency situations, it can cause ascending paralysis from the feet to the face including the heart and lung muscles requiring blood pressure support or oxygen, and in the worst case, a ventilator to support breathing. There are theories about the cause, such as a viral infection or immunizations that trigger the immune response.

Nurses are not known to be good patients and I was no exception. I was given a bed alarm after I tried to get to the bathroom by myself but instead ended up on the ground. Bed alarms are usually given to the elderly who are confused and are not safe moving around on their own. This would be an embarrassing memory I would relive during the quiet middle of the night moments when sleep would evade me. And then there was the bathroom incident.

I was feeling great one day in rehab. My nurse had left me in the bathroom to do my hair and get ready for visitors. I was on cloud nine. So close to discharge and feeling great. I could stand on my own, if only for a few minutes. It was during one of those vain moments that I turned too quickly from the mirror and landed on the bathroom floor. I couldn't get myself up. The best I could do was to struggle over to the corner of the bathroom so that I would go unnoticed as nurses walked back and forth in the hall.

Lucky for me there was a new patient needing everyone's attention. I was forgotten in the bathroom and all I needed to do was hide long enough for my friend to show up. I'll never forget the sound of her heels as she hurried down the hall. "Do you think you can get me up?" I asked. It took two tries, but she hauled my paralyzed body off the floor and into the wheelchair.

Three weeks after I was admitted to the hospital, I returned to work.

You probably know someone that has a diagnosis of autoimmune disease. More than half of the medical commercials on TV describe treatment of one disorder or another that is related to our own immune system attacking our bodies. There is no one magic bullet and many diagnoses, but the various diseases have too many similarities to ignore. Whether it be related to stress, weather (lack of sun), diet, a virus, or lack of exercise, autoimmune means our body decides to revolt and attack.

A nurse practitioner I've known for years recently asked me if I really believed I caused my own illness, and I said yes. Whether that was rational or not, I did believe I ignored my health and worked my body into the ground. I was a nurse and had seen so many examples of caregiving gone crazy yet ignored my own symptoms and felt responsible for the inevitable. I had the knowledge at my fingertips. I knew what mismanaging stress could do. It wasn't my intent to hurt myself, but the sheer ignorance in believing that I was somehow beyond sickness took its toll.

In *Denial*, Ajit Varki scientifically proves a theory first conceptualized by Danny Bower. What if humans evolved because of their power to deny reality? Humans may still exist because they learned to understand risk and immortality, the only drawback being they live each day anxious of the next bad thing to come. In the book, Varki mentions humans also selectively deny aspects of reality that we don't appreciate, like eating too much, drinking excessively, or not exercising. It's possible that denial can be routine enough that you risk your health, or massive enough to change your life.

I didn't stop long enough to question if getting back to work so quickly was the right thing for me or those I managed. I was avoiding the truth, so sure that my determination and desire to be back would surmount physical limitations. I remember feeling horribly anxious about what was going on at work while I was away. There were decisions that needed my attention. There were people covering for me that already had too much to do without me dumping on them. I couldn't stop myself from entertaining the thoughts that repeated in my head. *Finally, they're going to figure out they don't need you.*

The evening before I left rehab, I found it difficult to calm down because my friends were coming to visit. I was still in a wheelchair and remember being embarrassed that they would see me this way, so different from the biking buddy they expected. Instead, when they all arrived I felt nothing but gratitude and planned to start thanking them one at a time for their support as soon as I got home. I was overwhelmed seeing all of them together again, laughing while sharing old stories. I was going to get stronger, head home, be a better friend, wife, and mother. I had dodged a bullet and would take better care of this body that had sacrificed so much. Finally, I would be the woman I was meant to be.

Many optimistic thoughts churned in my head, but the thoughts that were the loudest and kept repeating like a broken record were as familiar as a best friend. *You are to blame for this. You had many chances to wake up, to find balance in your life, to be more present with your family.* As grateful and hopeful as I was, doubt that I would change, even with the huge wake-up call, surfaced.

The truth at the time was that I didn't want to choose any other life than the one I was living. There was a significant reason for my desire to stay in a job that was harmful to my health. I wanted and needed everyone's approval, not only from colleagues or from the hundreds of people I had managed, but from strangers too. I was a nurse and mom who cared for everyone else first, that's what I believed. I didn't have time to take care of myself.

I would remind myself about the promises I had made and my desire to change, then find excuses. I was procrastinating and hiding from reality. I began to blame my husband – after all, I had to keep working because I didn't have a choice. If he was a better provider, I would be able to stay at home and then I would be happy. Blame is a horribly insidious creature that will steal your hopes. Once you embrace it, strangers like anger, hatred, and disgust come to visit.

I was starting to feel like a character in a Stephen King novel. The deep dark secrets I kept to myself, the lies I fabricated, the horrible new thoughts I entertained morphed into lumps and bumps that started appearing all over my body. I tried to cover them up with more make-up and bigger sizes of nice clothes, believing no one else would notice I had been consumed by a *Jabba the Hutt*-like creature, now 70 pounds heavier than I had ever been. The power to deny reality, apparently a superpower all humans possess, can have a poisonous outcome.

This is life, full of choices, mistakes, and endless chances to be better every day. It will always be a process, life lessons absorbed over time, habits formed and hard to break. I did figure out how to balance my life, to find a way to sort the multitude of crazy thoughts swirling in my head, but only after I crashed, and this is what I want to share with you.

Maybe you've experienced something similar – a moment where you were forced to see how the stress of caring for others exhausted you and caused you harm – and you began a plan to take better care of yourself. Maybe you tell yourself that even though you've seen others get sick or burned out, you'll be fine; you'll figure out how to balance it all.

I eventually did learn the reasons why I wasn't making good decisions and then began to practice one lesson at a time. In the next chapter, we'll get started on our journey to finding balance by learning the process that's not only helped me, but many others. Knowing that we're hardwired as Nightingales to think of others first, learning what happens when imbalance becomes life, then, coming full circle to finding meaningful work can be a beautiful journey to embark upon. Let's pick a road and get started.

Chapter 3

# Spinning Your Wheels

*"In the end, only three things matter: how much you loved, how gently you lived, and how gracefully you let go of things not meant for you."*
**–Buddha**

Have you ever found yourself stressing about things that are beyond your control, or making things up to worry about? Do you find yourself unable to stop spinning your wheels, stuck in the never-ending chaos that is your life? Do you know what you're *spinning* about, sometimes looking around and realizing you are the only one stressing and everyone else is telling you to just relax? Like that's so easy!

The definition of *spinning your wheels* reads something like "busy doing nothing, making no progress, in neutral position."

21

This seems a negative way to describe what I had known as thinking. Spinning allows time to work through the details, to stress over them, and then finally, to decide to move forward. If I worried too much about how much time I was wasting with the process, I suppose I'd have one more thing to be stressed about.

While stuck in the process of spinning, I learned to look back which helped me to move forward. Being in neutral position can be comforting so long as you understand what's being offered to you in that moment in time. In the following chapters, you'll find the ten lessons I've put into practice from years of spinning my wheels.

But first meet Diane, a nurse who described herself as an overachiever with no boundaries: "I feel as though I live to work, but without making a conscious choice. I spend more time working than enjoying life. When weekends come, they fly by so fast and before we know it, it's Monday and it's back to work. How do we focus less on work and more on life and what's important? The balance you were describing is the goal. I always feel that what I'm doing is not good enough. Like I could do better, achieve more. It's exhausting. Never satisfying enough. Seeking perfection which is unachievable with so many opportunities that we want to conquer. Does this make sense?"

This type of stress is self-imposed for Diane and for many of us that believe we'll never be good enough and there is some model of perfect we haven't quite reached. If we were just a little more organized, started the day earlier, and worked harder, life would be more balanced. The real issue is not something others put on us; it is our problem to figure out. It's the constant drive to be the best – or perfect – and in the end, a deep fear we'll never get there. We spin our wheels as we question our careers, believing we're fulfilled but knowing we're not, and then wondering what and if we can do anything about it. This need we have is hard-wired and we believe impossible to stop, especially when our thoughts and actions spin out of control.

From one soul that *desires perfection* to another, there might be comfort in knowing that perfection is just a word, impossible to achieve, but nonetheless a powerful thought that repeats in our heads. We do have the ability to understand what the underlying issue is when we're spinning out of control, worrying about too many things at once. But that isn't so easy when you're caught up in the moment and find yourself unable to think straight. I use a method called *SPIN-IT* to help at those times.

I began the book with Marie whose favorite memories were of the many cycling trips she had taken before I met her. The visions of the colorful places comforted her. The gathering of beautiful people at a wedding, the somber faces carrying a casket from a small village church, the deep burgundy-colored pasta sauce, the shiny gelato, and the orange-leafed vineyards became companions she frequently brought back to life.

I could easily recall my own visions of breathtaking countryside from the seat of a bike. The perspective while pedaling down a quiet road is so different than from a car or bus, the spinning of wheels sometimes so thrillingly fast that there was only joy in my mind. Other times, the wheels spun painfully slow when the grade of a mountain forced more struggle and my internal voices were the loudest. It's in the slow spinning of the wheels that the thoughts come alive, with ideas that inspire one to dare to live differently, but lessons can be learned from crazy, wild spinning too.

There are different degrees of spinning, from the quiet digestion of thoughts to the chaotic chatter that could be described like spinning a car out of control and crashing. There are times when spinning can make you first feel lighthearted, then dizzy and off-balance, like being spun into the air as a child or twirling barefoot on the grass during a hot summer night. There are times when spinning can make you throw up, like my sister did all over me on the *Spider*, a gut-wrenching swing ride at the carnival.

Regardless of the type of spinning you relate to, there are lessons to be learned. It's possible to put the dreams into action one spin at a time no matter how out of control you feel, no matter how unlikely it seems that you can slow it down. Even if you believe your life is already spinning too fast and you have no choice but to continue the ride no matter how sick it makes you, you can find a way.

In the following chapters, you'll read stories covering each of the ten lessons in my life course called W.O.R.K.L.I.F.E., B.F.D. The lessons will consider Worth, Opportunity, Respect, Knowledge, Limitation, Inspiration, Faith, Exposure, Balance, and Forgiveness with a concluding chapter on Desire.

We reach for the stars that seem just beyond our grasp; we want results now and get impatient when they don't immediately appear. We're dreamers, this group of Nightingales that find pride in their hard work. So imagine what our lives could be like if we were to work as hard to live our wildest dreams? The training program includes WORK, four lessons that teach you to *spin*, LIFE, four lessons that teach you to practice journaling – the art of the *simmer* –allowing time to digest and stew over past experiences and finally, BFD, three lessons that teach you to put a plan in place, to *soar!*

## W. Worth: Know thy self-worth.

Who defines your worth? What experiences young in life become the framework for our own definition? How do prior experiences set you on a path that either diminishes or enhances your worth?

### O. Opportunity: Learn to look opportunity in the face as a stranger first!

Does this opportunity fit for me or for who you want me to be? Does this sit well with me? Why am I proud of what I do, or why not? Are you stretching or shrinking?

### R. Respect: Pay homage to the young woman whose reflection seems familiar.

Write about the first time you were proud of your own accomplishment. When was the last time you experienced unrestrained joy like a child? How do you find those same experiences today? What are the ways you respect your body?

### K. Knowledge: The past, like the foundation of a home, supports expansion.

There is at least one experience in your career that challenged you physically and mentally, pushed you beyond your comfort zone. What did you learn from the experience? How did that experience change your life? In what ways could you continue to learn from the experience?

## L. Limitation: Inner lizards will hold you back. Learn to embrace the butterflies.

Are you friends with the voices you entertain? Are they only the positive mothering kind or are your voices the mean bullying kind? Who do you listen to the most? In what ways have your fear voices held you back? What are you afraid of? When was the last time you felt embarrassed?

## I. Inspiration: Inhale sweetly as if it was your last breath and be inspired!

When was the last time you did something creative? Can you remember the way it felt? What does creativity mean to you? How do you become inspired to act differently? What happens to your creativity when you're exhausted or distracted?

## F. Faith: Believe in the good of those around you; seek faith and advice from within.

Now that you've learned to entertain the voices, are you ready to practice reworking the message? Do you trust your ability to sort your thoughts before acting on them? Do you do what others tell you even when you doubt their advice?

## E. Exposure: Find comfort in vulnerability and celebrate authenticity.

What if being exposed was the new thing, no longer a weakness, but a fad everyone followed like low-waist jeans? When did you last feel naked? What are your most sacred desires that you don't share with anyone? Are you living an authentic life? What is holding you back?

## B. Balance: An unequal load on either side tips the scales. Once tipped, balance is harder to achieve.

What have been the tipping points that caused you to lose balance? How do you determine if your job is right for you? Is work your life? How do you maintain balance while you do the work you love?

## F. Forgiveness: A forgiveness ritual is critical to loving yourself and others!

Make a list of the thoughts you will forgive yourself for entertaining. Do you believe you deserve forgiveness? What do you have to let go of from your past to move forward?

## D. Desire: Practice a kaizen-like method to achieve your desires.

Do you desire to live a more balanced life? In the conclusion of the course, you will identify solid steps to begin your own life plan.

**SPIN-IT** refers to a process that allows you to change the way you manage your thoughts, or how you respond to someone during a conversation. The process forces you to pay attention to your thoughts or to what is being said to you by others, consider them, then rethink and state out loud a new thought. It can be used to coach yourself through old patterns to provide you with the opportunity to change how you react. When used to coach others, you offer a very effective way to guide them through the same process.

**S = Say your thought out loud (or restate what someone else has said out loud).**

**P = Pay attention to the thoughts now spoken as words. Evaluate.**

**I = Investigate by asking yourself if the thought is true, validate it (or investigate further if you're coaching someone else).**

**N = Now, restate with care. Ask for help.**

**I = Internalize (or confirm if coaching).**

**T = Tell the new plan (or seek acceptance if coaching).**

By following the lessons and practicing the *SPIN-IT* method, you'll have the opportunity to reflect on moments in your life that were transitional and to understand how you managed the changes that took place. You'll learn more about yourself and the reasons you've accomplished so much in your life and why that still doesn't seem good enough. You'll explore your hidden talents and what brings you joy and inspires you. And finally, you'll set a plan to live the life you imagined.

Overachievement is a superpower many of us required to succeed in managing our hectic lives. Much like superheroes, there is weakness associated with any strength. It is in our belief system as superwomen who can do it all that working harder and juggling more will get us to that perfect balance in life. Our poison, like Superman's kryptonite, is the loss of so many special moments that zoomed past us while our minds – full of crazy thoughts – kept us constantly searching for more.

I lost my balance and fell many times, literally and figuratively. I couldn't walk for a while, then learned to balance my body on two shaky legs, then to take timid steps again, one numb foot slowly in front of the other. Then I learned to climb up stairs and turn around and look down again without losing my balance, then to begin the descent – the scariest thing I had ever tried. It was in learning to walk again that my perspective began to change, and I looked forward to the struggle of climbing mountains again, slow as a turtle – who won the race anyway. Let's take your first steps together!

*Part One*

# WORK

*"Let the great world spin forever down
the ringing groove of change."*
**–ALFRED, LORD TENNYSON**

*Chapter 4*

# Worth

*In youth, it was a way I had,*
*To do my best to please.*
*And change, with every passing lad*
*To suit his theories.*
*But now I know the things I know*
*And do the things I do,*
*And if you do not like me so,*
*To hell, my love, with you*

**–Dorothy Parker**

## Lesson 1 – Worth: Know Thy Self-Worth

Who defines your worth? What experiences young in life become the framework for our own definition? How do prior experiences set you on a path that either diminishes or enhances your worth?

We are all shaped by the experiences that hold the strongest memories and force the most powerful thoughts. To find a fulfilling career that allows you to remain centered and to move forward without feeling stuck in your thoughts, you must be clear on why you're paying attention to those that might be holding you back.

In lesson one, we will explore self-worth, because without it, you won't understand why you've allowed yourself to ignore your biggest wants. With a strong sense of self-worth, you will serve others more effectively, finding peace in a career that fulfills you. We've all heard love will not find us until we first love ourselves. Without first finding balance through acknowledging the importance of self-worth, the ability to care for others will absolutely fail – even if it takes years to happen.

The definition of worth in this context is the value someone is rated by others but more importantly, how one views themselves from another's lens. Self-worth is the value one places on oneself, a reflection of how we see ourselves and judge our own actions. We learn about human value from a very young age. In the quiet observations of those around us, we gain an understanding of acceptance and denial, sometimes by words and actions, sometimes in the reflection from the eyes of the beholders. There are moments in our lives that make us question whether we are more – or less – deserving than anyone else. Can you remember the first time you knew your place – the first time you saw your value reflected in the eyes of someone you loved? Is that same value reflected in the mirror?

When we meet someone for the first time, we ask, "What do you do?" As in, what is your work – what do you do for a living? The question assumes work is how you *make* a living but for many, it also reflects your value or worth. What if we had to answer the question, "Who are you in this world?" I'm not a philosopher or a psychologist, but let's consider that question for a minute.

I do place value, a tremendous price, on the work I do, to the point that it's often very difficult to be anything else. But who am I in this world besides that? I am a daughter, college graduate, nurse, wife, mother, coach, mentor, friend, lover, perfectionist, business executive, cyclist, middle-aged woman, cook, jewelry designer, seamstress, dreamer, and sometimes a liar. It's true, I don't always tell the truth. I hide the truth from myself and from those I care about. There might be prettier words to describe it, but any other would be the same as paint on pigs.

We are all made of complicated body parts, nerves, and brainwaves that work in concert to allow us the opportunity to adapt to try new things and to determine our own set of beliefs and values. Work held the highest value in my complex make-up because of the positive attention I received from the many people who had become a substitute family and because of the amount of time I spent working and away from home.

I cared so much about pleasing others that I became distracted and less focused on those who really loved me: my family, my husband, my children, my friends. Those same people didn't get the real me. I was so focused by the desire and need for attention that I closed myself off, hiding from the people who loved me, creating this other person that sought approval from people I barely knew. What did I know about being authentic, being a wife, a mother? Did I fake those parts of my life too? I didn't even know the answer; I was already so good at pretending.

Karen Moning said, "The most confused we ever get is when we try to convince our heads of something our hearts know is a lie." I have lied to my heart. I have convinced myself over and over that what I was doing in this world fulfilled me and for several years, it worked, until I couldn't face myself or the lies I continued to tell.

Denying the obvious transitions that pull us in life and refusing to move forward for fear of change can be the worst kind of deception. I had a place in this world and I belonged, then I refused to move forward despite the huge changes at work that I couldn't stand. I had the signs right in front of me but was afraid of what came next – so comfortable in the skin of the hack I had become – so used to the paycheck and the security.

Laurel was stuck much like I was. She wanted to make a change but was scared to do anything but what she was used to. Laurel was 47 at the time we worked together. I asked her to describe being raised by her parents, about her childhood. She was raised by very young parents and always remembered how hard they worked to feed her. Her young impression was that they were gone from the house for hours at a time working and then they would come home and make dinner.

"They seemed so tired," she said, "but they didn't ask anything of us until we were much older. They wouldn't have noticed if I had sat on my butt all day. I could have but I didn't. I was the third in line, not the first-born son, not the first daughter, and for as long as I can remember, I worked as hard as I could for my parents."

"Try to think back to your first memory of working. Where are you? What are you doing?" I asked.

"I was five I think because I remember coming home from school. We had moved to a new town and I loved the house we lived in. Outside, next to the house, we had a fenced yard with a playhouse and I was there a lot. I liked being alone and I took care of the house, cleaning, and sweeping the floors with my little broom."

Laurel was finding her place. She was watching and learning that hard labor was valued in her family. And once she was older, her playhouse make-believe cleaning became a real effort and her parents noticed. She said, "As I got older, I started doing things around the house that they noticed. Once they started commenting, I couldn't stop myself. I became the cook and the maid in short order and I liked it."

No one asked Laurel to do the work, there wasn't a chores chart with bright shining stars in the kitchen, no allowance, so why? What motivated her to cook and clean the house after school as she became a young teenager? "I can remember from a young age feeling responsible for the burden I placed on my parents. Another mouth to feed, more messes to clean up, how overwhelmed they were. I wanted to help, clean the house, do the laundry, wash the dishes, cook ... anything that would make them see I was useful and necessary," she said.

Laurel continued to work hard into adulthood and had success in her career. She was offered promotions because her managers noticed her efforts, and the attention boosted her. She was proud of her accomplishments, but over time she began to question why she was still so caught up in the work, why she couldn't say no and why the voice that said *you hate this* wouldn't be silenced.

Her self-worth was completely tied to her career and the people she had known for almost twenty years. The nagging thought that it was no longer enough was frightening. Despite her best efforts to ignore the changes coming her way by working even harder, she doubted she could sustain the pace. *If not this, then what*, she thought?

Know thy self-worth is the first lesson in gaining the strength to move forward. Laurel thought she knew herself and the place she held in this world but began to realize she had created this other person that was all of the things she did. She was a daughter, college graduate, wife, mother, etc. Some of those things she accomplished on her own, with hard work, while the rest were the many normal responsibilities a woman accepts.

Instead of the question, "Who are you?" we must ask who we want to be now.

Laurel's work ethic began more than forty years ago, when she first realized it pleased the most important people in her life at the time. It served a purpose and became the reasons for always saying *Yes* when asked, always wanting to make people proud. Because she did make people proud, she became more confident in her roles, but less aware of what *she* wanted.

*"Who are you?" said the Caterpillar. "I-I hardly know,*
*Sir, just at present," Alice replied rather shyly, "at least I*
*know who I was when I got up this morning, but I think*
*I must have changed several times since then."*
- LEWIS CARROLL

We are the thoughts we pay attention to, so which *worth* voice is your best friend, your inner lizard, your confidant? It takes practice to learn which voices should get most of your attention, but let's assume that you are among the majority who find it easy to entertain the worth-*less* thoughts. There is one voice that is the captain of your shame team. Let's call her Sophia Shame-On-You – Sophia SOY for short.

Sophia SOY is always right there, waiting for her chance to let you know how you screwed up. Her team says things like: *You're nothing, who do you think you are, you're a fraud,* and *I told you so.* And because you've known her and the shame team for so long, it's hard not to listen and to believe, deep down, what they're saying, especially when you're already feeling bad, stressed, or exhausted. *SPIN-IT* gives you a quick process that allows your more supportive voices to be heard.

Sophia SOY and her team will always be a part of your thoughts, but you don't have to act on their advice. Let's use *SPIN-IT* to practice turning the negative upside down.

- S – What did you *say*? Say it like you heard it.
  *I heard you. You said, you're such a loser.*

- P – Pay attention, entertain the thought.
  *I'm a loser? I've thought that a lot. I remember when I really screwed up but it turned out okay.*

- I – Investigate with a question. Do I really believe?
  *Do I really believe I'm a loser? Am I going to choose to live with this thought?*

- N – Now, restate with care. Ask for help.
  *Sophia, I have listened to you and have trusted you, but not this time. You can't distract me. I need confidence right now.*

- I – Internalize and restate.
  *I am not a loser – look what I've accomplished, I am a rock star, and I can do this.*

- T – Tell what we're going to do.
  *We are going to go in there and make this happen. Let's do this!*

What value do you place on your worth as an individual in this world? There is no one else like you. All the worth-*less* thoughts that spin in your head are just that, worthless. But without the ability to slow your thoughts and address them individually, you might just find it difficult to listen to the one voice that needs your attention. The combination of inheriting the Nightingale gene – to be constantly tuned in to everyone else's needs – and a confused self-worth, thinking other's needs are more important than your own, is a set-up for living off balance. Know and love thy self, first, then serve others.

# Chapter 5

# Opportunity

*"We have to get used to the idea that at the most important crossroads in our life there are no signs."*
**–ERNEST HEMINGWAY**

**Lesson 2 – Opportunity: Learn to look opportunity in the face as a stranger first!**

Does this opportunity fit for me or for who you want me to be? Does this sit well with me? Why am I proud of what I do, or why not? Am I stretching or shrinking?

To maintain balance in one's life, developing a sense of skepticism before venturing into a new opportunity is important. In lesson two, we'll explore why nurses might make decisions about career advancement that will add more work and stress to their lives. While promotions can have a significant impact, both financially and personally, understanding the real reasons one jumps in to quickly add more work must be understood. One might arrive at the same answer – to take the offer – but we'll learn why holding off and doing more soul searching is always a good idea first.

There was a time when I said yes to every opportunity that came my way, regardless if it was the right thing for me to do. I didn't question myself – if someone important to me suggested I do it, I did. My mom suggested I get my certified nursing assistant license because the community college was offering it to high school students, so I did, and that decision made a big difference in what came next. I learned a lot in the emergency room and on the floor of the small rural hospital and the best part was that I was mentored by my own aunts and uncles who were nurses there.

The year was 1980 and I was being pushed by those very same relatives, my nursing instructor, and teachers to decide what I was going to do next. I had a year before graduation and it was time to apply to college. My dilemma was not what I was going to do but where I was going to go and what kind of degree to get.

I could do the safe thing and take nursing at the local college, be a two-year nurse and continue to work at the hospital while I was going to school. We had no money for college and this plan made sense. My family was divided, but I was paying more attention to my aunt than anyone else. She saw a different life for me. I was afraid of what she described to me, a place so far from home, a big city full of strangers. But I was terrified of staying where I was too.

She drove me four hours for the interview at Seattle University. She had researched the school and knew they offered a scholarship for young people (ninety-seven percent of all enrollees were women) who came from rural communities. Because I had a high GPA, hospital experience, and came from a rural community, I had a good chance of being accepted into the school and getting the scholarship.

I doubted her – but more myself and my abilities – the entire time. I wouldn't know for years how fortunate I was to have an aunt who had been out in the world, who saw and pushed me. There would also come a time when this opportunity no longer existed for women like me; it would become much more difficult to fund an education in nursing which would further limit the numbers of students from underserved small towns.

In 1981, the four year degree programs for nursing in the state of Washington were limited. The University of WA was determining acceptance by lottery because of the high numbers of qualified enrollees seeking a state education. My aunt's knowledge of the programs and her efforts to help gave me an option I would never have considered. I would have stayed and attended the community college. Instead, I graduated from SU in 1985 while working at Swedish Hospital as a student nurse for two years.

In Malcolm Gladwell's David and Goliath, I would have been who he described as the "big fish in a little pond." The hours I logged in high school working in the emergency room allowed me to gain hands-on clinical experiences that put me a step ahead of most of the students at SU. I became a student instructor in the basic nursing lab and had more access to the instructors and the lab because of that. I thrived in the smaller private college environment, but would have been swallowed up at UW if I had been lucky enough to be selected in the lottery.

The lesson up to this point in my life would not have been, "Look opportunity in the face first as a stranger." Charles Swindoll said, "We are all faced with a series of great opportunities brilliantly disguised as impossible situations." When you're young, there is the need to walk into situations with a sense of fear about the unknown while remaining open to the possibilities of what you can accomplish. Once you've conquered the fear, your opportunities become endless, especially in a field like nursing that is both expanding in need and withering in popularity.

Nurses are in demand and can play the field. Much like dating with Match.com, despite your best efforts in describing yourself and in researching your perfect match, there is still the first "stranger" date. Job hunting while career building can be very similar. They want you, you're the perfect fit, they'll sell you hard on the position, and it will sound like your dream job. And it might be, or you might just be wearing rose-colored glasses.

Like that first date, careful planning for job interviews is critical to landing the perfect career that supports balance in your life. Preparing yourself in advance – through self-evaluation of your strengths, then review of weak areas or challenges you avoid – allows you time to scrutinize the opportunity without falling in love too quickly. Given the nursing shortage that became more significant leading into the twenty-first century, a nurse with a degree could have any job she imagined, and some she'd never heard of, without much effort. The dating pool was suddenly very big, unless you were the one recruiting.

The Bureau of Labor Statistics stated in 2014 that by the year 2022, the nation will need to have produced 1.13 million registered nurses and advanced nurse practitioners to fill the jobs being vacated by those retiring and the increased demand for healthcare required by the baby boomer population. In 2010, it was estimated that roughly 10,000 baby boomers would turn sixty-five every day beginning in 2011 and that number would continue for the next nineteen years. The baby boomers account for twenty-six percent of the U.S. population and are approximately 79 million strong. The healthcare crisis we all read about is upon us and we're just getting started.

Healthcare companies that are service providers, not product manufacturers, are unique in both their ratio of female to male reps and in the high percentage of nurses hired to support patient and caregiver education prior to discharging patients. As the nursing shortage spread throughout the U.S., it was harder to find qualified and interested nursing candidates. Recruiting, interviewing, and hiring had once consumed twenty percent of my daily responsibilities, but in the past ten years began accounting for more than forty-five percent of my time.

I started to look opportunity in the face as a stranger first. You can learn to quickly scour a resumé for key words that stand out, not the ones that a resume builder will include for you, but words that describe interest (personal and professional), work history, work ethic, loyalty, flexibility, perseverance. Weeding out used to be part of the process, but with the shortage, networking and "selling" the company and the unique positions became more critical. We spent more time dating and courting, looking for the perfect match and trying to avoid the famous and damaging words, "It's just not a good fit" spoken within a few months of investing in the hiring and training.

The most sought candidates for positions within healthcare companies other than hospitals are nurses with a unique skill set of clinical and sales experience. The nursing shortage further limits recruiters in finding that needle in a haystack nurse willing and able to add sales to their resumé. These nurses have the right personality and drive for sales but also enjoy the hands-on patient education, the interaction, and clinical experience the positions offer. The hurdle – more like a seven-foot-high jump bar – is getting a nurse to accept the word sales in their job description.

Let's spin a recent conversation I had with Becky, an oncology nurse who was looking for an opportunity to get out of "floor nursing" and find work in a more flexible job. She said she didn't really know much about homecare, but liked what the recruiter said about the position offering new challenges and that every day was different. She had become bored with the daily grind and started looking on LinkedIn and Monster, but wasn't sure what she was looking for exactly. I applied SPIN-IT to her fears.

I asked Becky what about the position concerned her.

S: "I'm not a sales person. I am sure I couldn't do that! The thought alone scares the crap out me." (Say it)

I replied, "Becky, you might be surprised to hear that this comes up a lot during interviews. There is a difference between being afraid of learning a new skill and not wanting to because of the skill itself. We have impressions of sales people because we deal with them almost daily. You've probably had great experiences and horrible ones even on the same day. Say the first five words that come to mind when you think of a salesperson."

P: "Pushy, gross, dishonest, slimy, manipulative." (Pay attention, entertain the thought)

I said, "Those words describe our worst impressions of sales people and a lot of them have earned the stereotype. So, if I added to your earlier statement 'You're not a sales person,' you don't think you'd want the position because you're scared to death of being thought of as pushy, gross, dishonest, slimy, and manipulative?"

I: "Well, yeah. That doesn't describe me at all and I wouldn't want anyone to say that about me." (Investigate further)

"Becky, tell me about a patient that you had to force to get out of bed and take a walk. You know, the crabby one that would rather just stay in bed and get pneumonia than make a move? How do you get Mr. Jones to take a walk without yelling at you or trying to hit you?"

N: "I make a plan. I ask him questions first, because I'm not sure how he feels. I assess him while we talk about the day. I mention that I read his chart and he hadn't been up in a few days. I convince him that it's in his best interest to get up. I also talk about the risks if he doesn't start moving, Then I get a time commitment from him and his promise that the walk will happen before I leave my shift." (Now restate)

"Becky, you just ran through a sales process like a pro. I think nurses are highly qualified in sales. It's what we do every day and we do it naturally. There are different sales techniques, but we use consultative selling with patients and physicians every day. We first ask a lot of questions, followed by affirmation to make sure we got it right. Then we follow with what we can offer and what the risks will be if the offer isn't accepted. Then we confirm. Try it with me. I'm a patient going home and I don't know you or the company. What would you say when you come into my room?"

I: "Hi, I'm Becky and I work for the company who's going to take care of you at home. Is now a good time? Your doctor said you get to go home today and that can be scary for people. I'm going to walk you through what happens, so you won't have to worry, but first, let's go over a few questions I have. Then, before I leave, you can ask me more. Sound good?" (Internalize)

T: "Becky, you did great. Did you think you were pushy or slimy? You were helpful and calm. Patients do get really scared to go home. They're so used to having the call button and getting a nurse, but deep down, home is where they want to be. This position might not be a fit for you, but don't let the image of a gross sales person stop you from considering the job. Be open to the possibility that this position could be perfect." (Tell it)

There are many opportunities for nurses, young and old, given the healthcare crisis we face today. Finding the perfect fit is so important. Work is part of the balance equation and we must first seek to ask questions of the stranger that is a new opportunity. Have a list of great questions that force the recruiter or hiring manager to describe why you would find the job a perfect match. The number one red flag for me during the more than 10,000 hours of interviewing was if a candidate had no questions at the end of the discussion.

The same applies if you're looking to make significant changes in a career you've had for years. Careful thought and attention is required to make the decision to improve your work-life balance, to stay or to go, and finally, to determine what exactly is causing the chaotic thoughts in the first place. What if you were to develop a list of questions for yourself, much like an interview for a new position? Some questions I've found helpful include:

1. Tell me about what you love to do when you're not at work.
2. Why, in this stage of your career, are you looking to make a move?

3. What about yourself makes you a good candidate for a new career?
4. What stopped you from making a career change once you knew you weren't engaged?
5. What thoughts hold you back from supporting this necessary change?
6. What are you afraid of, the fear you don't say out loud?

Before deciding to accept a new opportunity, protect yourself by looking carefully at what the change will do to you and your family. A new job adds stress and uncertainty which can further impact balance. If you are in the position of managing a team, these same questions apply to candidates. Answering the questions listed above can help you sort not only why you're thinking of making a change, but also if it's the right one. Understanding the importance of finding work that supports balance is your primary objective.

Chapter 6

# Respect

*"All that we are is the result of what we have thought.
The mind is everything. What we think, we become."*
**–BUDDHA**

**Lesson 3 – Respect: Pay homage to the young woman
whose reflection seems familiar.**

Write about the first time you were proud of your own
accomplishment. When was the last time you experienced
unrestrained joy like a child? How do you find those same
experiences today? What are the ways you respect your body?

We start out young and hopeful, full of confidence that
we can do and be anything we imagine. As we get older, we
make mistakes and spin on thoughts that force regret. Soon,

doubt nags, even with the simplest of tasks. To find a more balanced life, we must first understand the question, "Do you cherish the woman who stares back from the mirror?" In this lesson, we will work to answer the question, because without first acknowledging what you've become, it is impossible to find your way back to who you want to be in this world.

*I promise to respect my body and to stay healthy and physically fit for you,* was what a childhood friend vowed to her husband to be on their wedding day. That one sentence has stuck with me for more than twenty-five years. I didn't give my body a second thought, not then and certainly not for many years following. I was already married with toddlers which came fully equipped with exhaustion and eating whatever was left on their plates.

Looking back, I think my friend was intuitive beyond her years and protective of herself. How could she have known at such a young age that respecting your body should be at the top of the list of life promises? I don't remember when I first began to dislike myself or when I first lost the sense that I could accomplish anything, but I do recall the very recent moment when I realized I hardly recognized the woman staring back in the mirror.

I had taken youth and strength for granted, the passage of time stealing the young woman I remembered being only yesterday.

Joan Didion wrote, in an article for Vogue in 1961 on self-respect, *"Once, in a dry season, I wrote in large letters across two pages of a notebook that innocence ends when one is stripped of the delusion that one likes oneself. To live without self-respect is to lie awake some night, beyond the reach of warm milk, phenobarbital, and the sleeping hand on the coverlet, counting up the sins of commission and omission, the trusts betrayed, the promises subtly broken, the gifts irrevocably wasted through sloth or cowardice or carelessness."* Joan described the beginning of the many lies she told herself and others and the subsequent piling on of guilt that would become a brutal effort to resolve.

"When was the last time you felt unrestrained childlike joy?" I asked Diana who was challenged by deciding what she would do next. She had accomplished so much in her work, but was questioning whether to stay in her position as a nurse manager or find something more fulfilling. Issues with retaining nurses and the constant training required once she found candidates was beginning to grate on her nerves. She was too young to officially retire, but was pulled to do something fun and rewarding before she did.

"I remember my aunt who was our babysitter when I was six. She was going to be a beautician and practiced on me. She had make-up bags full of tiny Avon sample lipsticks. She would do my hair and let me try the lipsticks while the Beatles played on the record player. I loved her fake red hair and mini-skirts and how she made me feel special. That is the last time I remember feeling like a kid. She died less than a year later in a car crash, when she was eighteen. Lipstick and music were my last favorite memories of her. I didn't know what to do with the feelings I was having, I was so sad. I didn't get to go to the funeral, I didn't say goodbye. I began to hide away in my room. Seemed like the only option that made sense then."

Is it possible, like Joan stated in her article, that there is a moment in our lives when the vision in the mirror changes, the moment when you first begin to slowly morph into someone you dislike? You begin to take on adult responsibilities and sometimes make the wrong choices, then to doubt yourself. At first, it's easy enough to ignore-possibly even deny- that change is taking place and the innocence of childhood is slowly fading.

I have to believe in the unrestricted power of denial, and my super power of procrastination. Because without either one, I am at a loss as to how I would explain why it took me five decades to take a hard look at the woman in the mirror and to admit I hardly recognized her. Little white lies, colored truths, and innocent exaggerations begin to build up silently like plaque in arteries, until there is no turning back.

Lack of courage leads to zero self-respect. Little moments – when you are called to be courageous, but fear takes the upper hand and you back down – become small little chips in your armor that over time rust and erode, opening you to the damage that lies will do, like the damage the winds, rain, and sun will impart from overexposure. I was given signs along the way that life is short. I wasn't blind to the path I was taking, I just chose to put the real me on the back burner.

It took bad accidents and a serious illness to force me to be fully aware of my own mortality. Then I became grateful that I was still here. I promised to live better, to take care of my body, to not waste another minute regretting anything, to spend more time living with intention. I wish a promise, a plan, or a want was that easy, but just like everything in life, we choose to spend time doing the things we want to do, even if for a moment we were appreciative and believed we were granted a wish to live differently and did for a second. What an extravagant waste to ignore the opportunity to change over and over.

I had formed the habits a lifetime ago and they worked for me as I accepted the promotions that were offered every time. I was successful beyond my dreams, at least that's what I told myself alone in my hotel room far from home. "If you had the chance to go back and offer advice to your younger self, what would you say?" was a question asked during the retreat. *You will be challenged as you grow older, but be brave enough to believe in yourself. If you take time, you'll remember moments when you found courage. When you face questions that scare you, stand up to what you know is right, even when your stomach twists in knots and even when you can't breathe. Pay attention to the voices that will point you in the right direction, but know that it won't be easy without practice.*

When I used to feel embarrassed, the first thing I would do was to get out of the situation as fast as possible. Fight or flight would kick in and I'd feel like I was in danger, so I would run. The thoughts I was listening to that created action included, *they know you're a fake, did that just come out of your mouth, what is wrong with you?* There is the opportunity now, at this moment to stop yourself, to choose not to entertain the voices that for years have demanded your attention. Instead of being on auto-pilot, trust yourself and the years of accomplishment. Have the courage to face the fear, change the thought, and finally, the action.

As an exercise, try the SPIN-IT method to consider your most exposed moment and how you reacted. Walk yourself through the thought that you were paying attention to – the one you couldn't ignore – and try changing it. What I've learned about the passage of time is how easy it is to forget that perspective changes like the seasons. A choice you made or something you did long ago that damaged your self-respect will look very different from the vantage point years have given you.

This is the one chance you get. It doesn't matter if you're a genX, millenial, or baby boomer. There are no do-overs. So, take a good look in the mirror and be courageous, and respect will follow. You can be successful as a hack, but so much more alive as the person whose reflection you barely remember in the mirror.

Chapter 7

# Knowledge

*"To acquire knowledge, one must study;
but to acquire wisdom, one must observe."*
**—MARILYN VOS SAVANT**

## Lesson 4 – Knowledge: The past, like the foundation of a home, supports expansion.

There is at least one experience in your career that challenged you physically and mentally, pushed you beyond your comfort zone. What did you learn from the experience? How did that experience change your life? In what ways could you continue to learn from the experience?

In this lesson, we begin to consider events from our past that supported the changes and decisions that led to what we do today. Taking time to look back at what was going on at that time in both your personal and professional life when you chose to make a change can be enlightening and well worth the exercise of reflection. Positions held – whether bedside nursing, management, or leadership – and your own life experiences set the stage for where you find yourself today. Until I took myself out of the daily grind, I was not capable of slowing down long enough to consider the past, to move from spinning out of control to thinking clearly about what could come next.

The women's leadership retreat in Hawaii, so far from my stressful life, allowed me to quiet my chaotic mind long enough to visit the many memories that held a special place for me. I revisited the ones that I cherished because they described someone else, before I almost lost everything that mattered, before I recognized the young girl staring back in the mirror. There were successes and many proud moments in my work life that kept me engaged but also torn as I found myself drawn to memories of family and friends, the places we had gone, the experiences we had known, and the children we had raised.

I've tried to account for the time I spent working, away from home, family, and friends. Why would anyone, if they had a choice, spend more than half of their adult life away from those who loved them? I'm comfortable knowing some of you are out there, judging and considering my sentence. Surely there should be a punishment for a woman more interested in a career than raising a family. There is nothing you could say that I haven't already told myself, almost daily, in one form or another, over the past twenty-five years.

Ten years ago, I didn't regret any of the choices I'd made. I was thrilled to be accepted, taking on more responsibility, and ignorantly soaking in the enormous stress that went along with the titles. I was high on my job and fueled by the excitement of managing my staff, consisting of over seventy percent women, mostly young and eager Nightingales. I was working in healthcare and believed I was helping patients and families experience illness in the comfort of their own homes by teaching them to be independent. My job felt meaningful.

Every year, we would perform employee satisfaction surveys. We would review the results and form small work groups to address two or three issues identified as most critical – in other words, the areas the employees scored as having the highest need for improvement. In the twenty plus years of managing a team, work/life balance was always in the top two.

Despite efforts to improve year over year, my team followed the low national averages. Recently I asked for confidential feedback because what I had done for years wasn't working. But did I really believe I was responsible for how my team managed their time? Everyone worked long hours and weekends. This was not an eight-hour job. The patients we cared for were so sick, requiring a lot of our time to get them safely home. It was the rewarding job we all signed up for, but not everyone on the team was on board with that concept. I thought I supported them anyway.

One employee was the most critical when answering the question of whether her manager supported work life-balance and I'll always be grateful, despite the bruised ego I felt for weeks following the survey. I struggled with the question because I didn't believe a company had control over how I balanced my life. I was fully aware that I gave a disproportionate share of my time to work, but that was my choice. My life was my work. I was proud to be responsible for the development of this young team, and was gaining confidence along the way.

At the same time, I was deceiving myself that balance existed in my life. I believed all my relationships were just fine, that I could love my job and equally love and be present for friends and family. I was organized and smart enough to juggle it all, and most of the team was independent, requiring very little of my time. Yet, here was an employee telling me I wasn't handling everything so great and that I negatively impacted her work-life balance – not the company, me.

The team I managed was growing quickly and the work along with it. I found myself working more often, stretching the hours, putting out the fires, then emailing late into the night or on the weekend so that the team would have direction or answers to their questions when they woke up. I was often surprised by how many would answer no matter what time it was, or whether it was on a weekend. I would *reply all* because doing so would mean one less thing to respond to later.

While I did not expect responses after hours to emails or for anyone to take a call on the weekends, I was sending the wrong message repeatedly. By acknowledging those who did respond, I was inadvertently sending the message that after hours and weekends were not sacred time for my employees. I was rewarding my *look-alikes* for working as hard as I did and essentially ignoring the ones trying to have a life.

Although the employee who gave me the feedback left shortly after, she started me thinking. I was ignoring a bigger issue, leading this team into the ground expecting the imbalance to be something one could get good at, like an ultra-marathon. Those who don't train hard enough or have the stamina eventually fall off the back in any endurance sport. I knew burnout was one of two reasons people left, that and management. It was time for a new retention plan.

There are some things a manager in healthcare has control over and some they don't. Understanding what drives nurses to stay or to go is a critical first step when putting a plan in place to retain strong employees. Nightingales serve others and find it very difficult to say no when asked, so burnout is a significant factor. Finding ways to minimize, not promote burnout, is a good place to start. Nurses cite several reasons for seeking employment outside the hospital, and those same reasons apply to homecare and outpatient clinic jobs as well. The most common reasons they leave:

1. Management: Poor communication, no team culture or vision and lack of attention
2. Burnout: Forced and unplanned overtime, short staffing, inflexible schedules
3. Fear: Safety concerns, too many patients, floating to other units, hurting someone
4. Disrespect: Management allows physicians to be abusive and to bully nurses
5. Salary: Not commensurate to workload, no perks, picking up extra shifts to earn

There are nurses working in hospitals that stay for years and some interesting programs put into place to keep them content. Of the fifty hospitals I reviewed, there were similarities in the programs that led to job satisfaction and employee retention. Some require an investment, but in one study, it was estimated that every nurse lost costs just under $100,000 to replace. In a 600-bed hospital, the estimated annual costs associated with RN turnover were six million dollars, so putting into place a retention plan that includes some financial perks had some payoff. The bottom line is that if nurses are not happy and healthy, patient care and satisfaction will suffer.

Nurse-friendly hospitals in the U.S. do some or all of the following:

1.  Financial incentives: tenure awards, pension programs, relocation, free counseling for staff and family, referral bonus when finding new employees, tuition reimbursement, sign-on bonus, nursing school loan forgiveness, home loan

2.  Foster team culture: interdisciplinary team involvement, grow-our-own mentor program, nurse center for professional development, advancement, job share

3.  Innovation: job sharing, telecommuting, simulation lab for new nurses, flexible shifts

4.  Wellness: onsite childcare, high tech fitness center onsite, shuttle service, bicycle commuting rewards, $ incentives for wellness program, one-month vacation

5. Perks: free public transportation/parking, dry cleaning facilities, movie discounts, holiday bonuses, recognition rewards, elderly care, career guidance professionals

Picture a unit in a hospital or a clinic where the nurses, doctors, and staff work together to turn the hard labor of caring for sick people into a fun and rewarding experience. Imagine potlucks with music and breaks in shifts to work out, job sharing, simulation labs to develop young nurses faster, a place where tenured nurses mentor their own new graduates for six months before letting them fly on their own.

The possibilities of defining a new culture and creating a vision that empowers both young and experienced nurses are unlimited, but it will take training both managers and their staff to work actively together to create the change. The number one reason nurses leave is not burnout, but poor management. If you are in management, or considering it, this is something you *can* control and have the influence to change. Strong nurses will not wait around to see if your previous plans take effect unless they believe they have a voice in the decisions you make and an understanding of the vision you're creating together.

This is a lesson about acquiring self-awareness. We are the sum of the things we think and of the actions we take. You might wonder what one person could do to make an impact that would begin to change the course of this healthcare crisis. You can lead a team, work together, learn from history, and speak up. We can all learn from past experiences to create safer and happier nests for our Nightingales.

*"If your actions inspire others to dream more, learn more, do more and become more, you are a leader."*
**–JOHN QUINCY ADAMS**

Part Two

# LIFE

*"I'm always calculating what I want to do, who I want to be, what I want to accomplish. I don't need to worry about that. That's always on a slow simmer. The muscle I have to work on is being more present."*
**–CHRIS PINE**

Chapter 8

# Limitation

*"Caution is the daughter of circumspection, but she tends to outgrow her mother."*
—FRANZ GRILLPARZER

## Lesson 5 – Limitation: Inner lizards will hold you back. Learn to embrace the butterflies

Are you friends with the voices you entertain? Are they only the positive mothering kind or are your voices the mean bullying kind? Who do you listen to the most? In what ways have your fear voices held you back? What are you afraid of? When was the last time you felt embarrassed?

This is a chapter about fear and how certain thoughts we pay attention to will limit us. Some of life's greatest memories stem from conquering fear and embracing butterflies. You might have had experiences that you promised yourself never to repeat again, but if you can learn to push past the fear, you'll find anything you desire is possible. A perfect example of this is public speaking, the most common experience people who have tried it once wish to never experience again. But if that is part of your job, simply choosing not to work at improving by working through the fear, is probably not an option.

It took me five years to attend a GBS support group. I wanted to forget I was ever dependent on anyone and feared I looked weak. I felt relief that I had gotten better, but also guilt, the voices in my head acknowledging my own culpability in the crime. There were so many people who came to the meeting in wheelchairs, on oxygen, or using canes to walk. They had been diagnosed years before without the rapid therapies available today. Despite my issues – with walking down stairs, balance, and energy – I was one of the fortunate. I began to question why I hadn't done more in the five years following my big wake-up call. Why hadn't I made changes to manage the stress that continued to pile on, or rather, that I continued to accept?

You've already been introduced to Sophia SOY and her shame team so let's talk about Frankie Fear-A-Lot, FAL for short. Frankie runs the scare squad and is best friends with Sophia. Frankie does her job by pointing out the many risks that might be associated with trying something new while Sophia jumps in with examples of things that have already turned out badly to stress the point. It's a wonder we try anything new, so high the risk of embarrassing ourselves when we fail later. You might be in the group that finds it much more comfortable to play it safe, having already experienced your own fear team.

Eleanor Roosevelt said, "You gain strength, courage, and confidence by every experience in which you really stop to look fear in the face. You are able to say to yourself, 'I lived through this horror. I can take the next thing that comes along.'"

This year, I had the fortune of working with Tracey who had a terrible fear of speaking in public. She had been asked to speak in front of a nursing conference, thinking it would be okay since she was to be part of a panel discussion, not up there naked by herself for everyone to see. Tracey described in detail with a shaky voice that while she thought she was prepared, the other speaker began first and was giving her speech almost verbatim. Thoughts began spinning in her head, *what am I going to say now, I can't do this, I don't know anything…*

By the time Tracey had the chance to speak, she was so overwhelmed with the thoughts she had been entertaining that she became sick to her stomach, her heart racing, her face sweating, and her tongue so dry she thought she might choke on it. Tracey did get through the speech even though her self-evaluation was she had failed, and she promised herself she would never do that again. She kept her promise until this year, ten years almost to the day when she walked off the stage.

She had a request to speak to a group she really cared about and wanted to say yes, but she was scared. She knew the fear was holding her back. She wanted to improve her speaking skills so that if she decided to do this, she wouldn't stumble over her words. I asked Tracey to describe the worst thought she had listened to just before going on stage.

S: "I couldn't stop thinking that I had no right to be there, I wasn't an expert, and everyone would know that once I opened my mouth. The longer the other nurse spoke, the more I knew I was right. She was so calm and was giving the speech I had prepared! I knew I was going to fall on my face in front of 400 people!"

*Tracey, you were asked by a large nursing organization to talk about your program. Do you think they would have done that if they thought you were a fake?*

P: "No, I guess not. I was running a large program, the first in the country to manage sick patients outside of the hospital. I did know what I was doing, but when I got there and saw the huge crowd, I started freaking out. All I could think about was I didn't belong there."

*So, you were qualified, and it sounds like you had something to offer that crowd. They could have gone to another presentation, but chose yours instead. There was something reassuring you could have said to yourself before walking on stage. Try it, what could you have said?*

I: "Am I really a fake? Am I going to believe this? Do I know what I'm doing?"

*Yes! If you had asked yourself those questions, your brain would have answered, "No, of course not. I know this stuff." What happened before you hit the stage for the first time ever is you were afraid, just like we all are when speaking in front of other people. You felt butterflies because your fight or flight response in your brain kicked in and you listened to your fear voice. By the time you walked on stage, full berserk butterflies had kicked in. Your brain believed you were in real danger and your body responded as if something was threatening your life. It's no wonder you could barely get through the speech. And, this also explains why you're not sure you ever want to do that again. Now answer the question you just asked yourself, are you a fake? Pretend like you're giving yourself a pep talk.*

N: "Do I really think I'm a fake? No! How awesome is this that I'm one of two people asked to do this lecture. I know what I'm doing. These people came to listen to me talk about my program. They need me. I know it's scary, but I've been practicing for a long time. Something like that?"

*Exactly, your brain can only really handle one thought and action at a time. While you're giving a pep talk and asking your brain to take it in, your fight or flight instinct goes on the back burner. Instead of running from the threat, your brain has no option but to think about what you're saying or asking. It also helps to pay attention to what's really going on when this happens.*

I talked with Tracey about fear. There is real fear – like confronting a bear on a trail – and perceived fear, which kicks in any time we're asked to do something we've never experienced before. Fear is a survival instinct and happens automatically and without discernment. Based on previous experiences, that fear can be very small like butterflies in your stomach, or out of control and very uncomfortable like the berserk ones I described earlier. There are tips to managing fear so that you can move through any new experience or reset an old memory of a bad experience by turning your thoughts around. By identifying the thought and calling it out, you can move forward with a different plan.

I: I might say something like, *"Hello Frankie. I know you're here to keep us safe, but this is not one of those times. I need confidence right now to help me do the best I can. Thanks, but put yourself on mute please."*

*Finally, move into action by telling yourself how it's going to go. You've got confidence driving now, what might you say before getting back up on stage?*

T: "We've practiced, and this is going to go great! I'm going to be calm and confident. No time for fear with this one, this group is counting on me!"

Thoughts are just clouds passing by in the sky. Sometimes we might see one that looks dark and ominous and start thinking about getting caught in a storm. We begin to pay attention to that one dark cloud even though the sun is shining through the rest. Our thoughts will limit our possibilities unless we learn to manage them and pay attention to the ones that will move us forward.

As Eleanor Roosevelt described, facing fear can be a powerful confidence-builder. Learning to embrace the butterflies and push past fear will free you to act on the possibilities you've only imagined for yourself. My most impressive memories, the ones that remain vibrant and alive, have come from experiences that pushed me beyond the berserk butterflies. Do you remember an experience of your own that, at the time you were doing it, made you question if you would survive the butterflies? How colorful is the memory, even years later?

Chapter 9

# Inspiration

*"After all, we believe what we see. To be inspired by
another is to be reminded that what stirs us so deeply
about someone else is, in fact, possible within ourselves."*
–KATHY CAPRINO

## Lesson 6 – Inspiration: Inhale sweetly, as if it was your last breath, and be inspired!

When was the last time you did something creative? Can you remember the way it felt? What does creativity mean to you? How do you become inspired to act differently? What happens to your creativity when you're exhausted or distracted?

Despite what you might think, we all have a creation itching to come forth. Anyone who nurtures their creative side finds something that inspires them into action, whether you're a nurse designing jewelry, a home chef-wanna-be, a painter, or an author. If you're working in a setting that pushes your stress buttons and exhausts you, it's often very difficult to find the time or energy to create a space for your inner artist to play, especially if inspiration is required at work. Who or what has inspired us in the jobs we do? Who were the role models you looked to for guidance and, even rare as it might have been, inspiration?

Marie mentioned how much her trip to Tuscany changed her life. She had never experienced a setting that inspired her as much as Florence, but she was also forced out of her normal routine, not just for a day but over two weeks. Even though she took her work with her, she spent more than eight hours every day stretching herself beyond her comfort zone and because of that, found inspiration that kept her going for weeks after returning to her demanding work. Immersing herself into work more than full time, her mind often wandered back to Italy and she was inspired once again. Believing success at work equaled more trips to Europe, she was inspired to work hard and felt more energized just thinking about the next vacation.

The year after our own trip to Italy, we went to France on an organized cycling trip with another couple. The cycling would require climbing a part of the French Alps almost every day, like the professional cyclists do during the Tour de France.

Within a day, it was clear I had signed on for way more than I was physically capable of doing. The rest of the cyclists were not in the same shape and quickly took to the mountains, logging their times and congratulating each other as they came to dinner every evening. I hated them, mainly because they took my safety valve away, forcing the support van to keep up while leaving me behind.

Most days the four of us barely made it to the hotel in time for dinner, so exhausted and frankly scared to death of what the next day would bring. None of us spoke French and rarely saw the tour van as they stayed close to the strong riders, leaving the two old couples from Seattle to fend for themselves.

At the end of every day, the group met to review the plan for the next day which meant taking notes on the maps that were provided while the ride leaders described where we were headed. My training for this trip included short evening rides climbing hills, and longer rides on the weekends. By the third day, I began to struggle and was worried I couldn't do the trip, let alone keep up. I started to take my own notes on the map, not trusting anyone. If I was going to get lost, it would be on me. It was a running joke that full assignment of blame would go to the ride leader if the ride sucked in any way, but the thought of lying dead somewhere in the French Alps kept me from laughing.

Less than five miles into the ride, we had already lost the rest of the cyclists. At a fork in the road, we had to decide which way to turn and without colored jerseys in front of us, it was up to the one of us who made the best notes on the map. I was sure we needed to go left but was vetoed by the other three. Granted, I usually deferred to everyone else when it came to maps, so my argument was lackluster at best and I trusted their judgment more than my own.

We took a right and proceeded down the most beautiful canyon I had ever seen, the rock walls shooting straight up from the road with small colorful towns nestled right into the rock. There were bird houses in bright blues, reds, and muted pinks dotting the face of the canyon as we turned a corner into a mountain village. By the time we had enjoyed the ride down while taking in the artist palette of colors, we were all convinced we had taken the wrong turn. Our choice was to continue a large counter clockwise circle, or go back up the canyon.

The ride ended in the dark, rain pouring down on us while we continued to struggle to find the house. We rode over 100 miles and climbed more than 10,000 feet that day. We ran out of food and water four hours before finishing the day. When I was sure I couldn't climb anymore, a cute little old Frenchman took me to the top of the last mountain pass in his truck, no translation required.

I learned four valuable lessons that day: I learned to trust myself over everyone else first; my body could handle way more than I had ever given it credit for; there would never be another ride that I could recall so vividly; and finally, pushing through the fear brought me more inspiration than I had ever thought possible. I was no longer afraid of a new challenge, and began to imagine all of things I wanted to accomplish, especially at work, as I thought of new ways to inspire the team.

I had spent years as a coach and mentor, but what had I done with intention to inspire the entire team, to create lasting momentum? I began to think of inspiration as a motivator and made a list of everyone I could recall who had impacted me in a way that forced action. Many speakers had left me entertained following their thirty minute presentations, but very few made a lasting impression.

I knew the places and things that forced my imagination and motivated me to create, but what did the women or men do exactly that inspired others? Did they have anything in common? Why were some of them so brilliantly alive, so much so that I wanted to be like them and thought maybe I could? While each person on my list had unique qualities, there were four common traits.

1. **Story Teller** – Have you ever been so caught up by a story that your mind refused to wander and therefore you learned more in ninety minutes than in a week? And the story, but more importantly the teller, stuck with you for years? Several years ago, Connie Podesta spoke to a crowd of 1000 on the topic of personalities … blah, I thought, another psychologist to fidget through because going to the bar was not an option. When she began to speak, I was spellbound. She had the whole crowd laughing and completely engaged, but more than that, I have never forgotten her simple tricks to knowing personality types, told with comedy, but also how to quickly identify those types among strangers. It can be very difficult to read patients and families when you walk into their room to talk to them. Connie's simple tools changed how I approached everyone.

2. **Trail Blazer** – Every woman in business knows the book *Lean In* written by Sheryl Sandberg, but what resonates with so many? I was caught up with the imagery in her book, the meetings she attended and actively participated in with high level people, and the courage she found to have a voice among the suits that had become comfortable talking down or even dismissing women. But most of all, I found her to be

real: a mother who made mistakes with her children, a woman who had the same insecurities we battle, and a leader who sometimes doubted her abilities. There are those among us that we can dismiss as impossible to relate to simply for their brilliant minds, but Sheryl spoke as if her book was written for me, and I was inspired to take her advice to speak up and lean in more often.

3. **Calm in a Storm** – To be able to inspire a team to follow despite the hurricane of change and impending hard work they know they're walking into is a rare trait. Having the courage to deliver the bad news, like *our ship might sink*, in a calm manner is a maneuver that can be learned, but to make it so believable that the masses walk into the hurricane is not. B.F. Skinner wrote, "Chaos breeds geniuses. It offers a man something to be a genius about." The first nurse manager I worked for was fired after thirty years in the position, not because she hadn't performed but because she was expensive. The entire time she was going through this significant transition in her life, she remained silent and professional. Had others in the same boat not spoken up, no one would have known how she was treated. She had a job to do and that was to continue to lead

her team. Geniuses of calm lead in the midst of chaos and bring us out of the storm.

4. **Energizer Bunny** – I had an inspiring leader who always said she was a work junky. She was addicted to meaningful work, to a culture of servitude and assisting the sick. She always started a talk with the mention of the heroes among us, those silent hard-working people who never bragged and always thought of others first. Finding someone who seems to have the stamina of five people while also slowing long enough to pay attention to those she's leading is inspiring. Executives are taught the importance of being attentive to the masses, but it's a rarity to find someone who really means it, is genuine, and grateful at the same time, and who you know works harder than anybody.

Elizabeth Gilbert wrote in *Big Magic*, "I have never created anything in my life that did not make me feel, at some point or another, like I was the guy who just walked into a fancy ball wearing a homemade lobster costume." Breathe in, breathe out. The physical act of inspiration and exhalation keeps us alive. Fail, take a deep breath, and try again to imagine your next creation. The art of breathing and dreaming will continue until your expiration date, and the only thing that will hold you back is fear. We've learned how amazing life experiences can be when facing fear, so what will you do next? Who inspires you to be your best self?

Chapter 10
# Faith

*"Working hard is important. But there is something that matters even more: Believing in yourself."*
–HARRY POTTER

**Lesson 7 – Faith: Believe in the good of those around you; seek faith and advice from within.**

Now that you've learned to entertain the voices, are you ready to practice reworking the message? Do you trust your ability to sort your thoughts before acting on them? Do you do what others tell you even when you doubt their advice?

Nightingales are not so great at having faith in themselves. You might think this doesn't apply to you, but it's in our very nature to serve and please others. It's not that we don't trust ourselves, rather, we're just in the habit of deferring to others. It's as if we had stopped exercising years ago only to be told to get up and run five miles. We're just out of practice.

I began to let the thoughts about my next move simmer on a slow boil that would last for days. *Should I stay? Should I go? What is keeping me from making the decision?* I knew the job had always been challenging, and some of the people I had to work alongside were more than difficult, but that hadn't changed and couldn't be the reason to go. Deep down, I wasn't onboard with the changes that pulled me further away from the intimate, meaningful job I'd become accustomed to doing. I was disengaged.

What was once a rewarding career had become something I disliked but what did that mean exactly? Why wasn't it enough anymore and who was I without it? The longer I stayed, refusing to take the questions on, the more I disliked myself for not having the courage to go, and the more my thoughts spun out of control. I was leading a team of managers and I had lost my way. The pressure to make a change before I destroyed them was overwhelming.

In a previous chapter we discussed how complicated it can be to hire strong nurses that fit well in today's healthcare environment. However, the most complex position to hire and manage in my experience has been the mid-level manager.

Management experience aside, screening for one's ability to make solid decisions in the heat of the moment with integrity takes a critical eye and patience. By far, hiring someone who lacks managerial courage will have the most damaging effect on a team. But again, it's the dating game. With a small pool of qualified candidates and plenty of competition *courting* the same, a frog can turn into a prince right in front of you.

Managerial courage is having the faith to do the right thing in the face of any challenge and putting your team's interests above your own. Even though in your gut you want to do something else because it's easier or because of selfishness, you are aware of the trap, you trust that you'll survive the fear, and you do the right thing. Over time, with confidence because of the skills you've developed to push past the fear, you stand out from the crowd of managers as a strong leader. I believed I had conquered this skill and was good at dealing with difficult people and the decisions that needed to be made, but lacked enough faith in myself to stand up and seek a new position. I wasn't even sure that was what I wanted to do.

Second guessing myself became routine and only added to the stress. This led to a change in how I made decisions. I began to exhibit a lack of managerial courage. I began to choose the easy path even though knots in my stomach told me not to (guilt). I always had an "exit strategy" and would be prepared with a story that justified my decision or someone to blame on the tip of my tongue. I gave in to this mode of management. I had listened to my fear team for so long, I'd forgotten what courage looked like. Frankie FAL had my full attention. She'd become my best friend.

Carrie, a manager of five years who had a higher than average turnover rate with her staff, asked me for advice. She wanted help because the open positions were having a negative impact on her numbers and overall morale was bad. She feared her job was in jeopardy if she couldn't figure out a new strategy to retain the strong staff she had left. I asked Carrie to describe her management style. "The team is really close. I have weekly calls where we do shout outs to the high performers. I know the team trusts me and will come to me with problems. I'm so close to them, I cry when they resign."

*You mentioned you've fostered a team that supports each other, trusts you, and they receive consistent recognition. Why do you think people are leaving the region?*

S: They're making mistakes. There's been so much turnover in the office that we're constantly apologizing to our customers about our failures. It's exhausting. It's no wonder that the team can't handle it. They start looking. I'm looking frankly – it's only a matter of time before I can't take it. I already quit once, but was promised things would change.

When you use SPIN-IT to coach, it's important to pay attention to find the one thing that stands out as the issue. In this scenario, "It's exhausting. It's no wonder the team can't handle it." Translation, I'm exhausted and I can't handle it and the team knows how I feel. *What do you love about your job?*

P: The people. I know they like me and I do a lot to help them. I only have a couple that need more attention; I'm not sure they will work out.

*Tell me about a time when you had to give one of them difficult feedback about their performance. What did you say?*

I: In November (six months before this talk) I had to write one of them up for being disrespectful to the staff. I mean, she's from the East Coast, so it's just the way they are. I wouldn't have done it if my boss hadn't forced me.

*How is she doing now?*

N: I just got another complaint from the office. She made someone cry, but her numbers are so good I don't want to say anything. It will blow over.

*What is the risk to the rest of your team and the office if she continues?*

I: I know I need to do something, but no one showed me how before you. It's not like I had training on this. This is the part of the job I hate. It will really screw up my numbers if she leaves.

*Even if you don't realize it right now, the team is watching you. They know this person is a problem and they see you ignoring the problem. What are you going to do?*

T: The next time she makes someone cry, I'll talk to her.

Carrie's lack of managerial courage was affecting morale and it's likely the reason she had so much turnover. Strong staff thrive with strong leadership and will not respect someone who lacks self-awareness and doesn't treat everyone the same. They will tire of trying to support this manager with boosts of encouragement. It's no wonder the team was exhausted. Issues that should have been simple to handle, like smoke, became as out of control as a raging fire. What once would have been easy to smother was now damaging everyone within vicinity.

Carrie's fear of being disliked kept her from doing the right thing and even with more coaching that involved role-playing to get through difficult conversations, she failed to accept that she needed to change anything about her style. Anytime we approached an uncomfortable moment, she pushed back and changed the subject, even becoming combative at times. This was clearly not the right fit for Carrie, but she needed the control and recognition to hide her fear and refused to acknowledge that this position was making her very unhappy.

Ultimately, it was Carrie's lack of courage to face the truth about her fears and inability to express her struggle that forced her decision to give up. Ambrose Redmoon said, "Courage is not the absence of fear but rather the judgment that something else is more important." Nothing was more important to Carrie than being right. Three other people left her team before she did, leaving a gaping hole in coverage and a detrimental morale for the rest.

Healthy balance takes many forms of faith. Faith that comes from outside – an unerring belief in something you cannot touch or see – becomes the North Star for many of us. Trusting in the good of others, that they'll do the right thing and have your back, is another. The first time this faith in others is tested and destroyed, one becomes a little more jaded, a little less likely to want to delegate, and then a lot more stressed in the end. The lack of the ability to rely on others and to relinquish control causes imbalance when the workload expected at the executive level becomes too much to manage alone.

Trusting yourself, putting faith first in your own best judgment while accepting advice from others can be tough if you've been raised to be pleasing, never objectionable, and always making others feel comfortable, even at your own expense. Habits develop to make decisions based on what others want you to do, trusting them first, judging yourself later. Small at first, the decisions begin to erode your confidence and you start to second guess even the most obvious right choices. The chaotic thoughts begin to surface, Sophia and Frankie leading the riots. *You should have, you can't, you won't, liar, fraud, hide me, take me away.*

I had to start planning. Spinning out of control was not sustainable and I could no longer do this job effectively. I made a list of the things I had to get done before I could make a decision to stay or to go, knowing this time, I wanted to make the decision that fit the person I saw myself becoming. Either I would leave the organization gracefully, with my head held high, or I would create the job that inspired me. I refused to walk away mentally before I had a solid plan and that included taking a leap of faith into my dream come true job.

- Join the Author Incubator (July 2017)
- Complete my first book (October 2017)
- Set a departure date (July 31, 2018)
- Review finances and set aside one year's salary
- Get a business license
- Complete a business plan
- Publish first book (January 1, 2018)
- Finish second book (February 1, 2018)

Ultimately, deferring to others to help you in making decisions can stall you and your ability to move forward. Have faith that you are the one most intimately involved with the voices you entertain, and the only one who can control them. I've taught you the method to begin to sort your thoughts in previous chapters. Another tool that will help you to be clear about what you want is to journal. I think of journaling as the art of cooking at a slow simmer. It takes hours to allow the food to change character and to ultimately develop complex flavors.

There is an art to journaling as well. Getting away to a quiet retreat helped me to slow down, and allowed me to develop the habit of free writing. Practice with some of the questions I've included so far in the book. Find a quiet place, preferably without music or other distractions, and allow yourself at least thirty minutes. Set the timer on your phone for three minutes and answer one of the questions. During this timed writing, avoid editing what you're writing or worrying about whether it's legible or makes sense.

Review what you've written and simmer on that for five minutes. Add to the entry if you want, or move to another question. Eventually, you will be adept at free writing for several minutes with very little effort. Finally, try journaling at different times of the day to see when you're most relaxed and when your inner voices are easiest to hear. Putting your thoughts to paper is an intentional act that leads to designing your best life.

Chapter 11

# Exposure

*"Don't be afraid to make things up.*
*Never fear being exposed as a fraud. Experts make things*
*up all the time. They're qualified to."*
–STEPHEN COLBERT

## Lesson 8 – Exposure: Find comfort in vulnerability and celebrate authenticity.

What if being exposed was the new thing, no longer a weakness, but a fad everyone followed like low-waist jeans? When did you last feel naked? What are your most sacred desires that you don't share with anyone? Are you living an authentic life? What is holding you back?

Oliver Cooper wrote, in his article on vulnerability, that there are many reasons one might not feel comfortable being vulnerable. Based on childhood experiences and sometimes reinforced in adulthood, there are true fears that limit one's ability to be authentic even if one wants to change. Some of those fears include memories that reflected heartfelt feelings such as being taken advantage of, being rejected, abandoned, hurt, humiliated, controlled, or betrayed. Creating a life plan that includes balance and meaningful work will require a reconciling with this question, "Are you hiding who you truly are because of pain you've experienced".

Authenticity requires vulnerability. "We cannot be our true self, if we are not willing to be vulnerable," Cooper said. Try to remember a time when your heart ached. What was the experience that led you to pull away from feeling that pain again? Being vulnerable can lead to a sense of empowerment and fulfillment, but letting go of past experiences has to be a first step.

The list was done, so why didn't I feel better? I had a plan and could visualize living my dream come true life. I would conjure colorful images of that life: a job I could control, my husband in our log cabin sitting in front of the cozy fire, trips to Europe, and cycling without the pressure of work taking up the space in my head. But the dreams only made my stomach aches and heart racing worse. I began to have trouble sleeping again, the thoughts like a huge audience shouting at a concert. No amount of tossing and turning would quiet them.

"Why are you so uptight, mom?" A question my daughter would throw at me at the perfect moment during the frequent arguments we would never be able to avoid, no matter how many times I said I'd never engage again. "Why can't you just calm down?" Good question. She knew how to expose the underbelly better than anyone else, maybe because she knew me best and could zero in on the issue even when I refused to admit it to be true. I have always been tightly wound like a Tasmanian devil wearing high-heels, running to the next thing that would allow me a distraction, an excuse to hide from what I was feeling.

In nursing school, we were taught the five physiological or basic needs of every human: oxygen, water, food, shelter, sleep. Maslow's Hierarchy of Needs – basic, psychosocial, and self-fulfillment – described a pyramid, with the most important need, the one that had to be fulfilled first in order to achieve the others, forming the base. Physiological needs, followed by safety were considered the basic needs. Love, belonging and self-esteem formed the psychological level, and self-actualization sat at the top. Only if physiological and psychological needs were met first could one achieve their full potential including the ability to be creative and to reach unlimited possibilities.

College rocked my sense of belonging, moving from a very small town where everyone was paying attention to what you did and where you had a sense of community that was solid. As a teenager, I started attending church with a friend, which reinforced love and belonging for me. Between school activities and church, I stayed very busy and spent more time away from home. I knew I was different than my siblings. We rarely spoke, except to fight – which made me want to hide out when I was at home, or better than that, spend as little time there as I could. But the first time I remember feeling truly alone was in college. Hiding my feelings became second nature.

I met great people in college, but wasn't very good at including myself in gatherings. I didn't belong here, I would tell myself. Who are these Catholic rich kids with credit cards and their own cars? I found my own community, others from far away, including four Vietnam vets who had to work to get through school too. They looked after me and reminded me of the uncles I'd left back home.

I hadn't been out of school more than three months when I began to think about moving back home. I had given up on finding a husband at the age of 22. Many of my friends were moving away and I began to isolate myself, going home right after work. Then, two months after taking my nursing boards and moving into my first apartment, I went to a friend's going away party. She, too, was leaving me to go to Ireland for a few months. I saw a man walking down the street in a red wool jacket, wearing 501s and carrying two chairs. My heart skipped a beat. I was carrying a chair too. *We must be going to the same party.*

The first holiday we spent together, having known each other all of eight weeks, started as an adventure we would never forget. We would retell the story during dinner parties, usually after being asked how we met. He was reading Shakespeare sonnets from a small blue leather book (seriously), while I was driving us to meet my family for the first time.

In the trunk and backseat of the car were about three dozen tins filled with beautifully decorated cookies, my holiday frenzied effort to bring joy home with me. This should have been a red flag of how anxious and *type A* I was to the man who would marry me. I always said, "He had his chance to walk away, right then or at least right after we figured a way to get out of the mess." He always said, "She tried to kill me and failed. How much worse could it get?"

I'll always remember the sonnets because truthfully, I might have been a little distracted by this man I already loved reading Shakespeare while I hurried us to meet the family, turning a corner too fast and losing control of the car. Black ice caused the rental car to slide like a bobsled over an embankment, the car settling between just enough alpine trees to stop us from falling all the way into the freezing creek below.

I totaled the rental car, and this should have been a sign to me since this was the second crash in less than four weeks on this same road, Honda Civic totaled in crash one, Buick in crash two. I would come to know myself as the years past. Accidents would happen to me when I was moving too fast, distracted by my constant thoughts and not paying attention. I guess you could look at it as the glass-half-full. If we'd been in the tiny Civic, he would have been right. I may very well have killed us both.

I remember feeling embarrassed in front of this man I wanted to impress but instead failed by taking us over a cliff. At least we only suffered bruises. His version of the story always includes the ransacked car, tins open everywhere with broken cookies scattered all over the back seat and trunk. Being the anxiety-ridden girlfriend soon to be wife that I was, I attempted to gather as many cookies as I could salvage into the dented tins, worrying about coming home empty handed, possibly more upset that my beautiful cookies would never be seen.

I may have been successful if it hadn't been for the noise that jolted both of us as we saw another car careening off the road, heading right for us. The shock and the look on his face made me realize I had gone beyond type A to crazy. I imagined my worst nightmare, not dying, but friends reading the story that would include the embarrassing truth:

*Seattle woman, 23, and her boyfriend, 28, crushed and killed by a falling car on Steven's Pass. Their bodies were found with evidence of colored frosting and sprinkles in their hair. It appears, while gathering broken cookies following their own car crash, they refused to move out of the way of the falling car.*

When he is the storyteller, I resist the urge to defend myself, embarrassed by the way it sounds...cookies? We do another dance, always during the holidays, when the flour begins flying around the kitchen, cookie cutters everywhere, colored frosting and sprinkles dotting the floor. He still doesn't understand why I get like this every year and I find it hard to explain. *It's Christmas. It's a tradition.* I was ignoring the signs right in front of me. "Why can't you just relax?" repeats in my head.

It might have been important to think of more meaningful traditions, like going away for the holidays with the two little ones who would be gone before I knew it. *Be careful,* he was trying to say. *This time of your life will be over, and you won't remember the cookies, only the years passing like cars on I-5 going 80 miles an hour – and the regret.*

Wasn't it enough that the cookie craze almost killed us? I know now that the holidays were always nerve-racking.

Marathon cookie making soothed and distracted me from the overwhelming anxiety I felt every time I got us ready to head back to my family, always searching for that sense of belonging and ignoring that it was right there in front of me. I barely knew myself when I became a wife and then mother. I learned that doing meant I didn't have to think about being and I became an expert at doing ten things at once while the years flew by.

Following thousands of interviews, Dr. Brené Brown concluded that the secret to strong social connection was vulnerability, not the act of being weak or submissive, but the courage to be your authentic self, to risk emotional exposure and the chance of being rejected. I hid from those I loved the most by busying myself with every imaginable hobby because I wasn't in touch with who I was. I isolated myself from a young age because I felt worth *less* than those around me. I knew pleasing others worked for me; it gave me a sense of belonging-false as it might have been-and that would become the way I functioned until I couldn't stand it any longer.

"Being vulnerable is scary, but is an inevitable part of social relationships. Opportunities present themselves to us every day; the question is whether we will take them," said Brown. Once I made the decision to change my life and began to face the truth, my hidden fears, insecurities, and doubts about my real strengths came crashing to the surface. I didn't know what to do with being so exposed, committing to being truthful no matter what the circumstance. Making stuff up was no longer an option if I was going to have my dream come true. I began first by being truthful with myself through journaling. The process was empowering and what I once thought of as a horribly embarrassing past experience, became more manageable and I was able to laugh about myself for the first time.

That was the gift of becoming vulnerable and accepting exposure. I have been uptight and anxious for as long as I can remember. It took giving myself a break and laughing about the obvious for me to relax just a little and to begin to learn to enjoy the ride.

Maybe you can point to a moment in time, or something that triggered a transition for you. Maybe you know in your heart you're not living up to your true self because of fear that you'll be lost in the process. The freedom lies in knowing you'll find your way to living the life you imagined for yourself, that the process won't be perfect but you'll get there, one step at a time.

Part Three

# BFD

*"Just try new things. Don't be afraid.
Step out of your comfort zones and soar, all right?"*
**–Michelle Obama**

Chapter 12
# Balance

*"I think for any artist, your voice is always evolving.*
*For me, the constant is finding a tension or balance*
*between drama and comedy."*
–LISA CHOLODENKO

**Lesson 9 – Balance: An unequal load on either side tips the scales. Once tipped, balance is harder to achieve.**

What have been the tipping points that caused you to lose balance? How do you determine if your job is right for you? Is work your life? How do you maintain balance while you do the work you love?

Finding a job that supports stress reduction in your life – or making significant changes in the one you have – will keep enough of the stress in check to tip the scales more into balance. Both work and life provide daily stressors that can be a healthy initiator for action, but for those who work hard but still think it's never enough, the pressure to put more on their plates can be a trap.

I had physical symptoms that would tell me when I was off balance, much like a fire alarm that might go off when a fry pan is left on a burner for too long. When I was consumed with work, I ignored the symptoms and pushed the limits. I ate and drank to dampen the loneliness, sleeping became a problem, and I was too tired to exercise. Work was my life. I could feel my high blood pressure in the throbbing headache that matched the beating of my heart. The more I worked, the more painful my feet and hands would get, so numb I would continuously rub them to stop the sensation you feel when your arm starts to wake back up from being slept on.

Then I would return home from an exhausting day and the look of my husband's concerned face would confirm I looked as crappy as I felt. He would rush me through the door and into a hot bath as fast as he could. Then I would feel guilty. I knew better and was harming not only myself in the work I was doing, but him as well. "I'm in this for the long haul. I love you and want you with me forever. You have to take care of yourself," he would plead.

Stress can be healthy in small doses when managed well. It keeps us on our toes and energized, but chronic stress – or stress out of control – has just the opposite effects. A job that is a good fit stretches you beyond your comfort zone, challenges you to continue to grow, while providing healthy doses of stress. Managed well, this type of job will keep you bouncing out of bed ready for each day with plenty of energy to spare at the end. The wrong one, however, can send you stressing out of control, so sure you can white knuckle your way to job satisfaction.

Every person experiences stress differently. What might be small butterflies that are excused away in one person will send another rushing to the bathroom, unable to differentiate stage fright from a real threat. The experience is so uncomfortable, they remember it, avoiding a repeat of the experience and missing out on growth opportunities that come along.

A job that forces this type of fight or flight routinely will cause unhealthy levels of stress. Paying attention to how you are reacting to the demands of your job and getting control quickly by developing stress-reducing habits that allow you to maintain balance can be difficult when the thoughts that get your attention push you to be better, do more, and work harder. The smaller voices trying to get you to take care, to slow down, and to live in the moment can be smothered.

I have learned that I was easily affected by the multitude of voices in my head (not the- you-have-twelve-personalities-trying-to-surface kind of voices, but a lot, some easier to recognize than others). It was like when familiar music plays softly, and you stop to listen because you like it, but then other loud noises – annoying ones like Sophia or Frankie's critical voices – fill the room and you've missed the moment to hear the soft melody. I call mine Maya My Own Respect Enthusiast, MORE for short.

In the movie *Men, Women, and Children*, at the beginning the satellite is slowly turning. It is clear you are above the clouds, above the sky you see every day. It is black, and there are stars and planets. It's beautiful, but you are distracted by the voices – people talking, static, the broken sentences that are clearer now. You listen harder. It's the whispers that you are trying to pay attention to, but the static is too scratching-on-the-chalkboard annoying to avoid, so you act without thinking it through, to get away from the disturbing feeling.

Maya MORE is trying to get your attention now. It is possible to have a job you love while enjoying the life you live. But it takes a conscious effort to sort the thoughts that drive you beyond what's healthy. Maya knows there are ways to relieve stress and how much better you feel when you are intentional about working toward balance. You get away to Europe, or take a long bike ride, or gather friends for a weekend retreat and work seems more manageable.

First Lady Michelle Obama said, "Women in particular need to keep an eye on their physical and mental health, because if we're scurrying to and from appointments and errands, we don't have a lot of time to take care of ourselves. We need to do a better job of putting ourselves higher on our own to-do list." How much more successful would you be if Maya (or your own respect enthusiast) became the main voice writing your to-do list?

Here are three stress relievers – besides getting a good night's sleep, eating right, and exercising – that can be incorporated into your daily routine: 1) Play – puzzles, games, a group sport like cycling – with your children, spouse or friend 2) Pets – get one, play with one, be around one. 3) Laugh – go to a comedy show, watch one on TV, gather with friends who make you laugh. While this seems reasonable, jobs that require a lot of your time, especially travel, can make finding time for daily stress relievers more difficult, especially if you spend a lot of time alone.

There are people that, no matter how hard they try to manage the daily hits of work and life stress, can't stop the accumulation of the hormone cortisol, leading to a chronic and unhealthy situation. Early signs of stress that warrant attention include inability to sleep, chaotic thoughts or strange dreams, aching jaw (from teeth clenching), inability to make decisions, weight fluctuations, increased sugar, alcohol, or drug intake, and headaches. Left unchecked, these symptoms can progress to migraines, hair loss, high blood pressure, drug or alcohol addiction, impaired immune system, and many other chronic conditions.

I agreed to work with Sarah who had left the hospital job she had for ten years for another because it was a great opportunity. She had regrets; the money was great, but she found herself more stressed than before and her husband and family were not happy with how much time she was gone. "I can't make anyone happy. The new job takes more of my time. I think about quitting all the time. I thought this job would be the answer." I asked Sarah what was the main reason she left her job.

S: I deserved more money for how hard I was working. They didn't appreciate the sacrifices I was making.

*Was it the money then? If that were true, with more money you should have been content?*

P: I thought I wouldn't mind the extra work, the kids could have more, we could travel more. I thought it was the money. I made a mistake.

*What would it look like to be doing what you love, Sarah? Imagine yourself in that moment.*

I: I love to cook. I would do that. But that's stupid. Cooks don't make any money.

*You're judging because it's scary. If you picture happiness doing something completely different than what you've always been good at, what someone else hires you to do, it can be terrifying to think about who you are if not that corporate woman who gets a pay check every two weeks. Turn the thought around, I love to cook, it's not stupid…*

N: I love to cook for people. It makes me happy to see everyone enjoying themselves, laughing, talking. Hours go by and I don't even notice. Cooking can't be stupid if so many people enjoy themselves because of it.

*Stupid is just fear talking. This is a big departure from your corporate life. If it were the smartest thing, the most responsible thing, what would you be doing?*

I: I would cook, at home or at a restaurant. I would write a cookbook.

*Your homework before we meet again is to begin to entertain these thoughts. Say them out loud, picture yourself doing these things that a woman does when she is an author of a cookbook. Try it. It's nice to meet you. What do you do?*

T: I just finished a cookbook. I took three months off and moved to Italy. I took the kids for the summer.

> *"Imagine life as a game in which you are juggling some five balls in the air. You name them – work, family, health, friends, and spirit – and you're keeping these in the air. You will soon understand that work is a rubber ball. If you drop it, it will bounce back. But the other four balls – family, health, friends and spirit – are made of glass. If you drop one of these, they will be irrevocably scuffed, marked, nicked, damaged, or even shattered. They will never be the same. You must understand that and strive for balance in your life."*
> **–BRIAN DYSON**

Is work punishment for you, or your passion? If punishment, why do you think that is what you deserve? What do you get out of it: recognition, belonging, security? The decision to make a change takes careful consideration to avoid the common pitfalls you'll regret later, if you take a new job believing balance is right around the corner because the grass is greener, the pay is better, or I'll be happier. Unless you address the thoughts that get your attention and dig deep for the reasons behind why you act the way you do in every job you take, you'll be right back where you started, and eventually spinning again.

Chapter 13

# Forgiveness

*"More than any of us, she had written her own story;*
*yet she could not wash it out with all her tears,*
*return to her victims what she had torn from them,*
*and by so doing, save herself."*
—SANDRA WORTH

**Lesson 10 – Forgiveness: A forgiveness ritual is critical to loving yourself and others.**

Make a list of the thoughts you will forgive yourself for entertaining. Do you believe you deserve forgiveness? What do you have to let go of from your past to move forward?

If you've hung in with me long enough to read the last lesson, you're probably wondering why it took me so long to get it figured out. I've learned to appreciate and give in to being older now, understanding better the many transitions and changes that can affect us all at different times in our lives and for different reasons. Losing my ability to walk and talk at almost fifty should have forced me to begin to live life differently, but I avoided the transition, unwilling to let go of my past, resisting the inevitable next phase.

William Bridges writes in his book *Transitions,* "Transitions in life's second half offer a special kind of opportunity to break with the social conditioning that has carried us successfully this far and to do something really new and different. It is also a time when we are surrounded by distractions. We're often still actively involved with our careers, and the house may not be paid for, the kids aren't done with college. Maybe we're coping with menopause or struggling across the burning sands of middle age." It wasn't likely the best time to be thinking about new beginnings, but I found myself energized and imaging the possibilities. Acting on those thoughts was the problem. I was incapable of taking the next step, no matter how much I thought about it.

Previously, I mentioned that embracing blame could invite other strangers like hatred and anger to visit. They didn't just visit, they moved in, as if they were in-laws demanding to be fed and loved. I did entertain them for years, coddling my anger like it was an Oscar for best feeling ever. I had a right to be angry. I hated feeling debilitated and weak. I resented my job for forcing me to continue the insane schedule. Nelson Mandela said, "Resentment is like drinking poison and then hoping it will kill your enemies." I wanted to want to be the person I was before I got sick, but I didn't have it in me. I had changed, and my competitive nature refused to give in to it. I was losing the battle but still hadn't admitted it to myself or anyone else.

At one point, still on medication for the nerve pain and barely keeping up with my work schedule, I got a call from my new manager demanding I take a flight to see him two days later. We had been arguing about my lack of attention to work. I refused to give in to his demands, but not because I expected him to know how sick I really was. I just said no. I excused him away because I had no respect for him – he should have known I was doing the best I could. But why would he have known, if I hadn't believed it myself?

I was miserable. I was disappointing my team and scaring my husband. I blamed my circumstances on everyone but me. These were the thoughts, the feelings I paid the most attention to. It wasn't the job I hated; it wasn't someone else that angered me. I knew what I needed to do years before I did it, and because I didn't have the courage to choose me first, I agreed to more work and piled on the stress and hated myself for it.

Byron Katie offers advice about not superimposing our thoughts onto reality, accepting that thoughts should be excused away, that what happens in the moment is what should be and is – nothing more and nothing less. "The more clearly you realize that would have, could have and should have are just unquestioned thoughts, the more you can appreciate the value of that apparent mistake and what it produced." Once I stopped spinning on what I should have done, what I did, why I couldn't, why it happened to me, and was it worth it, I began to move forward.

The thoughts I worked through with greatest attention focused on what I wanted to do next, what was possible for me, and how I imagined I would make it happen. By naming my strongest inner critics, I could sort them, address each for the efforts they brought to the table, and finally begin to quiet them to give confidence a chance to be heard. I began a list of thoughts I would forgive myself for holding and promised that once I repeated one on the list, I would turn it in a positive way before letting it go, never to be entertained again.

I forgive myself for:

- Shaming my body. *I am proud of how strong I have become. This is my body. This is me.*

- Failure. *My children are who they need to be right now. They were safe and loved.*
- Jealousy. *I am the sum of all that I have experienced and felt, no one else but me.*
- Cowardice. *I push past the fear. It is what has already happened. I am what's next.*
- Procrastinating. *I will do everything with one hundred percent conviction when I'm ready. It's time.*
- Dishonesty. *It's already written. I have nothing to fear of myself. Come out now.*
- Ignorance. *I will be open to a fresh idea from anyone or anything every day.*
- Scarcity. *I love and am loved. I will pay attention to all the beauty in this life.*
- Judgment. *What has already happened is. I do the best I can in the moment.*
- Blame. *I am in control of my thoughts and my actions. I am what happens to me.*

The art of forgiveness is the same whether you are asking to forgive yourself or another. The first step is to realize that *to err is human* and making a mistake does not make you a bad person, just a real person. Knowing you made a mistake and learning from it does provide room for growth as long as you're willing to forgive.

Asking forgiveness takes practice, especially if you've allowed thoughts about your self-worth and shame to confuse what happened. If you believe you really are bad and every mistake confirms that, you will lack the courage to apologize, further solidifying the negative thoughts about yourself. When you've ignored another's feelings by refusing to acknowledge a mistake, you know they know you hurt them, and every encounter without a sincere sorry becomes painful, escalating until you'd rather avoid them altogether than face reality. No time like the present works here; the longer you wait, the less likely you'll be to ever apologize.

Often, my apologies would sound defensive. I had already rehearsed over and over why I did what I did, how bad I felt, and why I sucked in general, and believed it. There have been times when I procrastinated so long, I never said I was sorry, confirming my beliefs that I was bad, I sucked, and everyone else knew it too. I would start spinning, as many of my inner critics would cheer from the rooftops, *"You suck, we all suck!"*

I learned what to do. I began to turn my thoughts around and became proactive at asking for forgiveness. My apologies were sincere and heart-felt. What was once sure to be a full-blown sweat-producing scene, played out with grace and eventually confidence.

S: I would like to talk to you about last night when I yelled at you. (Say it out loud)

P: You were probably wondering what you did to make me unhappy, but it wasn't you. (Pay attention)

I: You know what I'm talking about, right? (Investigate)

N: I'm sorry I hurt your feelings. I've been crabby lately because I haven't decided about my work and I took it out on you. I'd like to try again by explaining (Now restate with care and empathy in mind)

I: I have been trying to work this out and am getting frustrated. I could really use your advice if you're willing? (Internalize)

T: I was thinking I'd talk to my boss this week about a transition plan. I would like to hear what you think about that. (Tell it)

Here are a few tips to help if you've avoided these conversations in the past. Sometimes writing out the apology helps you prepare and makes you less likely to forget.

1. Take time to figure out what you did or said. Avoid trying to figure it out in the heat of the moment. If you are still uncertain what that was, ask.
2. Once you understand what you did or said that upset them, you need to understand why you did or said what you did. What is really going on?
3. Put yourself in their shoes. By imagining yourself in the same situation, you are more likely to feel what they feel. Example: If he had said that to me, I would have been angry. Without empathy, your apology can sound insincere, causing further harm to the situation.

Forgiving yourself and others can be a catharsis far greater than resentment or retaliation. It allows the memory of the wrongdoing, self-inflicted or onto another, to be minimized and even forgotten. This lesson was learned over time. I have forgiven myself for taking so long to learn what might have been simple for others. I learned to let go of the painful parts of the past, and the situations that embarrassed me, to seek forgiveness, and to move forward.

Chapter 14

# Desire to Do the Work

*"This is my life ... my story ... my book.*
*I will no longer let anyone else write it;*
*nor will I apologize for the edits I make."*
—STEVE MARABOLI

Do you desire to live a more balanced life? In the conclusion of the course, you will identify solid steps to begin your own life plan.

Nightingales are known for qualities that so many people admire: the ability to be open, trusting, caring, and compassionate. The work is hard, the hours long, and their priority will always be to care for others. Yet when out of balance, time may go by and, despite their best efforts, nothing changes. You might have thought the same many times. I can't stay, but what if I don't? You may have spent hours wanting a change, only to find yourself thinking the same a year later. Intention is the answer: not the want but the action. Until you have a plan, in writing that you refer to every day, even your best intentions will fall away. This chapter is about not only desiring a change, but doing the work to make it happen.

Nothing worth having is easy and I still doubt every day that I can sustain the changes without slipping back to my tried and true routines. After all, haven't I promised myself to lose weight, bike more, eat healthy foods, spend more time with family, and cook every day many times over the course of my life? The answer is that I can't do things the same way anymore and succeed. Knowing that deep down, I'm a perfectionist at heart, I set myself up for failure every time. I wasn't wired to do anything slowly, and my actions were a reflection of the chaotic thoughts spinning in my head. If I wasn't perfect, I gave up.

In the past, when I promised myself to lose weight, I'd start out strong. I would join Jenny Craig, or Weight Watchers, or do Slim Fast, or shoot myself up with HCG. I would buy new cookbooks and subscriptions to Self and Weight Watchers magazines. I would join a gym, buy a trainer, and work hard. I would picture the slimmer, better, stronger me and know I would be happy when…. The programs were always great at first. I stuck with them and felt high on the energy I was gaining, further cementing my commitment.

Then work would get in the way and I'd stay out too late and drink, then wouldn't exercise, or I'd miss an appointment, then I'd cheat, then I would miss another one because I couldn't face the scale or the woman writing my weight down because she would know I cheated. And the world keeps spinning and another four seasons fly by, and then I crash my bike and break my face, and then I get sick, and then there's menopause, and then ... so many excuses. I had to try something different and that started with learning why I thought the things I did that made me feel the way I felt that forced the actions that I would regret.

I heard about kaizen five years ago in passing when a CEO at a hospital mentioned they were using the Toyota method for streamlining their patient transitions from admission to discharge. The *what* method? Further details described the use of kaizen and Six Sigma to ensure continuous improvement and forward momentum, no matter how small the improvement, no matter how tiny the step forward. In fact, the slower, the better – because it was proven that for any significant change to occur and to remain intact, small changes over a long period of time were more likely to last.

Kaizen is a Japanese philosophy that focuses on continual improvement throughout all aspects of life. When done correctly, it teaches people how to spot and eliminate waste in all processes required to function productively. There are seven phases of kaizen and I tested them with two changes I wanted to make in my life – two that were causing me too much spinning. I wanted to lose weight and stop drinking alcohol, both opportunities I had failed to implement time after time.

1. **Identify an Opportunity**: I have made significant changes in my thought process this year. I want to challenge myself to lose weight and abstain from alcohol.

2. **Analyze the Process**: I had failed in the past because I thought too far into the future; I set myself up for failure by being too hard on myself. My expectations were not feasible.

3. **Develop an Optimal Solution**: I did my research and decided Whole30 was a reasonable approach. It was a thirty-day program which would keep me focused on one day at a time. The program did not allow weighing, so any fluctuations from day to day would not derail me. I wouldn't even know. And finally, no alcohol. Not because of the calories necessarily, but because the intent behind Whole30 is detoxing. I couldn't trick

myself into saying vodka or bourbon were low enough in calories to cheat.

4. **Implement the solution**: I started Whole30 the day after Labor Day and committed to the entire thirty days. A friend agreed to do it with me for moral support which mentally helped a lot. I was afraid of what would happen when I stopped drinking after more than a year of drinking every day. I was most worried that I was an alcoholic and this would confirm the addiction.

5. **Study the Results**: The program was a success in that I didn't cheat once, even when there were days when the stress triggers had me thinking about drinking non-stop. The absence of a scale removed the mental games that go along with weighing. I felt a lot better after day 14. The first two weeks, I had headaches and was tired which made me realize what crappy food and alcohol were doing to my health. I slept better, like the dead. I lost several inches and began to wear clothes I hadn't worn in months.

6. **Standardize the Solution**: Whole30 is a paleo plan on steroids. No flours, not even rice or almond. No sugar, not even honey. No soy. The foods I could eat, I really liked. I felt better without bread and sugar. I loved the recipes and the challenge of making my own ketchup

and mustards. I will continue to eat like this. I don't miss anything except ice cream, but this is a lifestyle change, not a diet. The change in that mindset has made it easier to sustain.

7. **Plan for the Future**: Every part of what I do now, I think in terms of small steps. I had a routine of setting myself up for failure by being too rigid and shooting for the moon every time, only to chastise myself later. From coaching to business planning and training, the small steps over time concept works.

"We cannot just survive anything goes. We can take control of our lives. We can quit sleepwalking. We can say right now, these are our lives. It is time to start living it. Whatever you do, pay attention. Let's bring soul and character to what is already there." More than 20 years ago, a fictional sports agent named Jerry Maguire wrote those words and more, in his heartfelt 25 page manifesto. His moral conscience was not accepted well by the very company that inspired the memo, which led to the loss of his job and all but one of his clients. In the end, Jerry pushes past the fear of having no money and no clients and puts his beliefs to the test. He began to live by his written word and attracted many clients who admired his compassionate and honest approach to their dog eat dog world.

While I'm not suggesting you write a manifesto to start your year, I do believe that taking the time to be clear about your values, beliefs, and desires creates intent. It isn't easy to take time to design a plan, even if making change is always on your mind. Life gets in the way. There will always be external forces distracting us, so the goal of designing a plan with intention is to allow yourself to be attentive to your instinctive drives, those values and beliefs that guide your sub-conscious. Even our best intentions to slow down, to focus on our personal goals and to stick to resolutions can get buried in the dirty clothes pile of our busy lives.

Identify 2-3 priorities you'll take on this year for yourself. They might fall under the family category, or professional development, or money. Try to stick to no more than three, and begin to practice habits every day to get you to that goal. For example, if you want to be more mindful of connecting with your spouse or significant other, you might practice a daily act of kindness or complement. Remind yourself with a sticky note in the car or at your desk.

The steps are here to implement, the lessons examples for you to review as you consider your own transitions, develop your own plan, and implement the kaizen way, slow but steady. Just like having a support system helps to encourage you every step of the way, I'm here to help. You have what you need at your fingertips, but as life gets busy and calendars fill, good intentions can take a back seat. Working a plan and staying accountable to your plan can be one more thing that causes stress and, without constant effort, it can be easy to slip back to old habits.

You have been hugely successful in your endeavors to date, but something led you here. The voices that wanted your attention are clearer now, telling you how much more peaceful life would be if you could learn to give yourself the care and compassion you have so willingly given to others. It is your time to act now. What are you waiting for?

Chapter 15

# Conclusion

I conclude this book the day before my 55th birthday. The *She is Relentless* retreat is taking place this weekend without me, but I am there in spirit channeling thoughts of transformation for the ladies on the beach. I fly to D.C. on my birthday, where I will finish this journey with the publication of this book. I committed to this a year ago and I stuck it out, sometimes scared and limited by doubt, most of the time sure I would give up just like all of the other times I desired a big change.

I have asked myself many times this year, what exactly made the difference? Why was now the time when my thoughts were not just the many voices I entertained and became comfortable living with, but confidants and advisors that became restless and ready for change? Why did I desire to finally stop spinning my wheels and move forward? I know that it started with intention.

I said I would do certain things a year ago, out loud on that beach, and they all happened.

I have come to know there was not one answer to any one question. The process started more than 10 years ago, with experiences that pushed me in this direction, sometimes unwillingly. The energy I spent chastising, regretting, and judging is now used to imagine all the possibilities for this last act because of the lessons I've learned. Sharing them with you has been a great journey and I end this with a final story about Nan.

Nan worked her entire life as a nurse, rarely moving from one job to another. She was the exception, very loyal to her employers even when the gift was not reciprocal. She recently began to experience a lot of stress and burnout but didn't believe she had any options. She thought she was too old for anyone to hire her and she needed to just stick it out, but deep down, she knew there was no way she could last another year. She would tell herself she could, she had to, but even the thought caused her more stress.

We worked through the thoughts Nan was entertaining. I'm too old to get a new job, no one will hire me, or I might retire early if I cut back. "What if those thoughts aren't true, Nan. Do you believe those thoughts?" Once we worked through the SPIN-IT method, Nan began to be hopeful, even saying out loud that she would be a strong hire for anyone given the limited number of nurses trained like her, that she deserved more money for what she did, and that she would begin looking immediately.

The power of intention, speaking out loud in the world what you desire, is a miracle to observe. Within one week, Nan was contacted by another company seeking someone with her qualifications. She went through a speed interview over the phone and was hired in a job that allowed her more time at home, more pay, and a renewed enthusiasm about her career. She was excited and energized again, no longer entertaining an early retirement.

To you, Nightingale, I hope you find peace and balance in life and learn to appreciate being in the moment. We are an impatient tribe, finding so many people to take care of and unlimited things to fill our time. I have found journaling helps to slow me down long enough to appreciate what I have and to really see those around me that have influenced my life in such a dramatically positive fashion.

There should be no regrets in this life, but that too is a flaw we share, as self-critics, so quick to punish. If possible, find it in your heart to share the patience and empathy you so readily offer those in your care to yourself first and love this one unique being, in all its beautiful imperfection.

# Acknowledgments

Thank you to my work tribe, young and old. You were my coaches, my team, my family, my friends. And gratefully, among you, a few shining mentors that guided me along the way, without force, into a life I only imagined.

Special thanks to Dr. Jane Peterson who humbly shared with me her gift of teaching by trusting me with some of her favorite patients. I was a better nurse because of the talented professors at Gene E Lynn School of Nursing.

To the Morgan James Publishing team: Special thanks to David Hancock, CEO & Founder for believing in me and my message. To my Author Relations Manager, Bonnie Rauch, thanks for making the process seamless and easy. Many more thanks to everyone else, but especially Jim Howard, Bethany Marshall, and Nickcole Watkins.

And finally, peace in life to Kris Plachy, www.sheisrelentless.com who walked me down the path to finding my hidden self.

# Thank You

I hope you enjoyed reading The Nightingale Gene. The fact that you've gotten to this point in the book tells me something important about you: you're curious and you're ready to explore the reasons you've made the choices in your work that have you living a life filled with stress and overwhelm. You're ready to experience clarity and sanity in your job, ready to take one step at a time to live the life you've imagined for yourself. You can answer the question, "Should I stay or should I go?" confidently once you take the time to understand what motivates you and to finally set a plan to make the right decision for you.

To support you in making that decision with confidence, I created the Nightingale Checklist just for you. It's a simple diagnostic assessment to help you get crystal clear about your current level of stress, the number of stress relievers you've employed, and the degree of burnout you're experiencing.

You can get your copy of the Nightingale Checklist by visiting www.spinsavorsoar.com

# About the Author

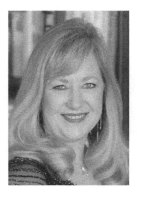

Jayne Van Brunt has a degree in Nursing from Seattle University. She has experience in healthcare management holding positions as Vice President of Sales and Corporate Sales Trainer. She uses the lessons she's learned about stress and living with a chronic illness to advise others. Her coaching and training programs help women in their efforts to find balance in their work and personal lives. Find Jayne at www.spinsavorsoar.com

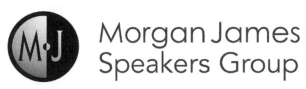

# Morgan James
# Speakers Group

We connect Morgan James published
authors with live and online events
and audiences who will benefit
from their expertise.

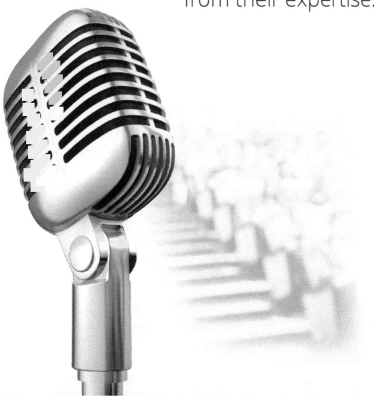

Morgan James makes all of our titles available
through the Library for All Charity Organization.

www.LibraryForAll.org

CPSIA information can be obtained
at www.ICGtesting.com
Printed in the USA
BVHW080358081218
535094BV00002B/6/P

9 781642 790269